ESSENTIALS
of the
NEUROLOGICAL
EXAMINATION

ESSENTIALS
of the
NEUROLOGICAL
EXAMINATION

BERNARD J. ALPERS, M.D., Sc.D. (Med.), LL.D.

Emeritus Professor of Neurology
Jefferson Medical College, Philadelphia

and

ELLIOTT L. MANCALL, M.D.

Professor of Medicine (Neurology) and Director, Division of Neurology
Hahnemann Medical College and Hospital, Philadelphia

F. A. DAVIS COMPANY
PHILADELPHIA, PA.

Dedicated to

L. S. A.

and

J. C. M.

Preface

This volume is a guide to the neurological examination as well as an inter-pretation of abnormal neurological signs and a description of commonly em-ployed ancillary laboratory techniques. In the course of his training the physician will have been taught the routine of a neurological survey. Further experience can provide increasing familiarity with the examination, as well as with an understanding of the central neurological problem. This manual therefore seeks to provide help for both complete and selective examinations, since it must be assumed that the doctor, for want of time, may be forced to perform a partial examination directed toward the chief or presenting problem.

Despite the fact that this manual is reduced to bare essentials, it should help the doctor in determining whether a neurological problem is present, what its location is, and how it should be pursued. A book such as this can supply only the basic facts on which to make a decision regarding the presence of neurological disease. Information as to its exact nature must be sought from other sources.

BERNARD J. ALPERS
ELLIOTT L. MANCALL

Contents

CHAPTER 1

Examination
of the Nervous System

An adequate examination of the nervous system is essential for even an elementary understanding of neurological disease. Unfortunately, such an examination is almost universally neglected among practitioners of medicine and is approached only with the greatest of trepidation even by students. A tap of the patellar tendons, a hasty appraisal of the response of the pupils to light, and a cursory evaluation of the hand grips all too often are looked upon as sufficient for most purposes. It is true that a proper neurological examination is a complex matter, but it is unfortunate that it should be regarded by most physicians as hopelessly beyond their reach and too obscure to be attempted except by the initiated. Such shrinking from an appropriate examination too often results in failure to recognize neurological disease, particularly if not far advanced. It is therefore of the highest importance to indicate to those who are not neurologists how to examine the nervous system and how to utilize the data so collected in a meaningful fashion. For this reason this chapter will be devoted to a description of the clinical examination of the nervous system itself; subsequent chapters comprise an account of the meaning and significance of the observations derived therefrom.

An examination of the nervous system requires systematic investigation of the mental state, cranial nerves, motor and reflex systems, cerebellar apparatus and of a variety of sensory modalities. For special purposes, investigations may be made of the autonomic nervous system as well.

In a general sort of way, both the history and the examination are directed toward determining, first, *where* the lesion is, and, second, *what* it is. If this approach is adhered to, many pitfalls in diagnosis will be avoided.

THE HISTORY

No examination can be complete without a history, and no history can be too complete. The diagnosis of any disease involves the careful collection and sifting of evidence; the taking of a history is the first logical step. The importance of the history itself is underlined by the fact that the diagnosis is often achieved primarily on the basis of historical data.

The recording of a history may follow two general lines: The patient may recite his story without guidance or help from the physician, or he may be guided in his presentation by leading questions. A proper history combines the two approaches. It is good policy to let the patient recite his own story and to follow this by pointed inquiries concerning pertinent points and information that may have been omitted. Any medical history is always better the greater the experience of the physician, a feature particularly true of neurological diseases. The greater the orientation in things neurological, the more pertinent and thorough will be the history. Despite this, much can be learned by aggressive curiosity and by the guiding principles that no history must be taken at proffered value and no symptom left unanalyzed.

All patients approach the physician with some degree of fear; hence their offer of historical evidence will vary with their own personality makeup. Some will make light of symptoms and offer little information; others will make too much of symptoms and offer confusing evidence; others will attempt to define their symptoms in diagnostic terms and by interpretations of their own; the rare patient will present his evidence logically and carefully. Because of the patient's anxiety concerning his illness his ability to recite his symptoms logically will be impaired. In this he will need the guidance of the physician.

The Family History

This assumes considerable importance under a variety of circumstances. It is of real significance in the spinocerebellar degenerations, in hereditary spastic paralysis, some forms of myopathy including familial periodic paralysis, in rare forms of peripheral neuritis, in amaurotic family idiocy and other neuronal storage diseases, peroneal muscle atrophy (Charcot-Marie-Tooth), Huntington's chorea, and in some forms of diffuse sclerosis. Migraine is typically a familial disorder, as are many instances of mental retardation, particularly those based on metabolic deficiencies. A familial incidence is found in occasional cases of multiple sclerosis, amyotrophic lateral sclerosis, and brain tumor. The occurrence of seizures in other members of a family becomes important in the diagnosis of idiopathic epilepsy. When a positive family history is obtained, an attempt should be made to delineate the genetic mode of inheritance.

The Developmental History

This becomes important in all cases of diseases of the nervous system occurring in infancy and childhood. Infections of various sorts may be transmitted across the placental membrane, while poor health in the mother may result in prematurity or inferior development of the infant. The health of the mother is of great importance during pregnancy, and great care is required to determine whether there has been evidence of avitaminosis, infection (rubella), or bleeding. Persistent vomiting, hypertension, and bleeding should all be inquired about specifically.

Particular attention should be directed toward ascertaining whether the child was premature or born at term. If premature, the exact details as to prematurity are essential. The duration and nature of the delivery should be investigated. Prolonged or precipitate delivery, natural or forceps birth are all important. The type of anesthesia and its duration should be investigated, especially in the case of barbiturates. The weight of the infant at birth and the condition on delivery are important, particular inquiry being made concerning cyanosis, jaundice, convulsions, and apnea. If initiation of breathing was difficult it is essential to know the duration of the period of apnea and whether intubation or the use of the respirator was necessary. It is important to know also whether the infant was breast or bottle fed and whether sucking either the breast or nipple was difficult or impossible. The rapidity of gain of weight should be looked into. Further developmental details concern the appearance of dentition; the age of development of sitting, standing, creeping, and holding up the head; the occurrence of talking; the development of toilet habits; the development of skilled acts; and in older children the school record and the occurrence of childhood diseases. Comparison of the patient's development with that of siblings is often of great value.

The inquiry into the development of the infant or child can be as detailed as one wishes to make it, but a bird's-eye sketch will suffice in most cases. No study of the development of the child is complete, however, without adequate inquiry into personality structure. It may become necessary to examine carefully the home environment with particular reference to the parents. Inquiry should be made as to whether the child was planned for and what the parents' preparation for childbirth was; whether there are other children in the family; what the personalities of the father and mother are, what their reactions are to the child, whether overprotective or otherwise; what the infant's routine is, and other pertinent features of personality development.

The Onset of the Disease

This is of major importance, since an analysis of the method of development of the illness gives important information concerning its nature. An abrupt or apoplectic onset of symptoms is found in cerebral hemorrhage and embolism, in some forms of brain tumor, in meningitis, particularly in the fulminating meningococcal form, in head injury, and in some viral encephalitides, to choose random examples. Even the time of onset of symptoms may be important, as in the early morning occurrence of cerebral thrombosis. The mere reporting of such an onset, however, is not sufficient. It is important to know, for the purposes of differential diagnosis, whether the onset was with fever, pain, injury, convulsions, or loss of consciousness. Acutely evolving paralysis of the legs with pain is something quite different from that without pain; in the former instance the orientation may be toward neuropathy or cauda equina tumor, in the latter, toward poliomyelitis or perhaps a parasagittal meningioma, to cite illustrative examples. Again, the occurrence of headache with fever suggests meningitis, systemic disease, or me-ningoencephalitis; without fever the orientation is totally different and suggests aneurysm, tumor, subarachnoid hemorrhage, etc. By careful analysis of such details it may be possible to obtain clues to diagnosis. It may also become evident on careful questioning that while the onset of the immediate symptoms was abrupt, signs of abnormality may have been present for a greater or lesser time before-hand. This is apparent, for example, in the history of high blood pressure and of transient attacks of vertigo or headache preceding the apoplectic onset of cerebral hemorrhage or with the transient ischemic attacks preceding thrombotic episodes. Disregarded headaches may have preceded the acute onset of symptoms of brain tumor, and pains in back or legs may antedate the sudden development of para-plegia in cases of spinal cord tumor.

In other instances the onset of the illness may be slow and the development gradual. In such cases one must determine whether the development has been steadily progressive or whether it has been broken by periods of complete or incomplete remission of symptoms. A slowly evolving disorder may extend over a period of months or years, and its beginnings may be so indefinite as to be lost in the past. Minor memory disturbances, increased irritability, mild personality deviations, all these may be so slight at first as to be disregarded, their true nature being apparent only when the disease has become well advanced. It is essential therefore that they be recognized early, a capacity that is possible only for a practiced eye and ear.

Progression of a Disease

The determination of the nature of progression and evolution of disease is also essential, since progression implies continued activity regardless of cause. It is important to know whether progression has been maintained steadily or whether there have been plateaus with stabilization of symptoms for varying periods, followed by more progression, or whether there have been remissions, more or less complete, for longer or shorter periods. It is equally important, moreover, to determine whether the progression of symptoms has been rapid or slow.

In senile dementia, as an example, the symptoms as a rule develop gradually and progress without letup. The same is true for most degenerative diseases, for some infections such as general paresis, and for many cases of brain tumor. Paral-ysis agitans, on the other hand, may develop slowly and progress gradually with interspersed periods of stability. A stuttering course with numerous clinical plateaus is often found in thrombo-occlusive disease involving larger arteries such as the carotid. In contrast, rapid progression of symptoms is found in malignant brain tumors, in amyotrophic lateral sclerosis, in some forms of general paresis, and in most viral encephalitides, to choose random examples.

The development of a disease with remission is of the greatest importance in proper orientation toward the correct diagnosis. It should be established whether remissions of symptoms have been complete or incomplete, and, if complete, the duration. The outstanding example of a remitting course is found in multiple sclerosis, but remissions occur in other diseases as well, such as general paresis, myasthenia gravis, some cases of brain tumor, and, rarely, spinal cord tumor. Recurrent symptoms clearing completely or incompletely are common in vascular disease of the brain.

The Nature of the Symptoms

When the method of onset of the illness is determined it is then possible to proceed to an analysis of the main complaints. It is essential to be on guard against taking the patient's word for any symptoms at face value. Careful analysis of the various symptoms of which he complains will help greatly in establishing a diagnosis. Thus, patients frequently complain of numbness of a limb or limbs when they mean weakness, or they may complain of dizziness without meaning vertigo in the true sense of the word.

Pain

The complaint of pain must be analyzed carefully. A complaint of pain in any part of the body should be analyzed along the following lines: (1) The exact location of the pain, and the path of any radiation; whether it is distributed along a peripheral nerve or has spinal root distribution, or along neither, as in central pain due to lesions of the thalamus or spinothalamic tract; (2) the duration of pain; whether it is constant or intermittent; (3) the nature of the pain with particular reference to its intensity (It is often difficult for patients to describe this feature of the pain, but a little patience will elicit helpful information. It is useful to know whether the pain is deep or superficial, lancinating and radiating from one part to another, or whether it appears all at once in all parts of a limb.); (4) the factors that relieve the pain; whether it is relieved by drugs and, if so, in what dosage; or whether it is relieved by heat, posture, climate, etc.; (5) the factors that aggravate the pain; whether movement, posture, climate, straining, sneezing, etc.

Headache

Similarly, a history of headache must be analyzed carefully with particular reference to (1) its location: it is essential to know whether a headache is generalized or focal, unilateral or bilateral; (2) its nature: whether it is deep or superficial, severe or mild, throbbing or aching, constant or intermittent, periodic or irregular in appearance; (3) its incidence; (4) the factors that relieve it; (5) the factors that aggravate it.

Convulsions

The problem of convulsions also requires careful analysis. In this connection it is important to determine: (1) The nature of the convulsion, with particular reference to such features as aura, generalized or focal characteristics, association with tonic or clonic movements or sensory disturbances. This information may be obtainable only from relatives or friends of the patient since the latter is usually unaware of the nature of attacks unless he has been informed of them. Petit mal or minor attacks, uncinate fits, motor or sensory jacksonian fits, and psychomotor attacks cannot uncommonly be described by the patient himself. (2) The association of loss or impairment of consciousness. This is an extremely important factor and one on which depend important decisions relative to diagnosis. It must always be inquired about specifically. If there is doubt as to whether it is present during a convulsion, the presence of a fall during the attack, or of tongue biting or incontinence will help greatly in reaching a decision. (3) The presence of post-ictal signs, particularly those of lateralizing value such as hemiparesis (Todd's paralysis). (4) The occurrence of the attacks, whether they occur chiefly during the day or in sleep, or both, whether they occur in relation to meals or with hunger, fatigue, or excitement, or whether they develop chiefly around the time of the menses. In this connection it is important to inquire into the spacing of the attacks and their frequency. (5) The onset of the attacks; it is essential to know whether the attacks have been present from birth, or whether they developed during infancy, puberty, or adult life. Inquiry should be made into development in relation to head injury, infantile encephalitis, meningitis, syphilis, hypertension, etc. (6) The response of the attacks to medication. Most persons with convulsions have had some medication before seeing the physician, and a knowledge of the nature of the drugs used and their effects is important.

Vertigo

Another symptom requiring careful analysis is vertigo. Most patients, even those of good intelligence, do not mean vertigo when they complain of dizziness. It is necessary therefore to determine whether true subjective or objective vertigo is present, the former consisting of a sensation of movement or rotation of the patient himself; the latter, movement of objects in the environment. A history of ataxia, nausea, or vomiting should be sought. Some patients use the term dizziness to indicate only a sense of faintness or giddiness or some nondescript sensation difficult to elucidate. Careful analysis of the complaint of dizziness will be repaid by a clearer conception of the disease in question.

Numbness

Another complaint requiring some analysis is numbness. It is necessary to define carefully what is meant by numbness; in many cases it will be clear that weakness of a limb or part of a limb is meant, rather than true impairment or loss of sensation. The presence of paresthesias, often tingling in quality, may be of material assistance in clarifying the complaint. It is of the utmost importance to determine whether the numbness has developed all at once in the affected part, whether it has progressed from one part of the limb to another, or whether there has been a march of the sensation, as in sensory jacksonian seizures.

Vision

A complaint of blurred vision covers a variety of meanings and must be looked into carefully. It may mean exactly what it suggests, but it may also refer to a variety of phenomena such as double vision, indistinct vision due to a scotoma, a sensation of blurring associated with a hemianopic field defect, or simply reduced visual acuity. All these can be determined by proper questioning. Diplopia especially must be analyzed carefully to determine if true double vision is present. Inquiry must be made in order to determine the position of the objects in relation to one another, the position of the false image, and whether the diplopia is present with monocular vision as is found in hysteria and in cases of local ocular disease such as retinal separation or dislocation of the lens.

These are but samples of the method of inquiry into specific symptoms of presentation in neurological disorders. They serve to emphasize the essential fact that no patient must be taken at his face value in the recording of his complaints. All symptoms must be analyzed carefully and in extenso in order to reach an accurate diagnosis.

When the history of the present illness has been completed, details of the *occupational, educational, marital,* and *past medical histories* must be covered in order to determine whether these offer factors of any importance in the illness. Not only must physical factors such as exposure to lead, arsenic, carbon disulfide, cold, and other hazards be investigated, but it is important as well to determine whether the work is interesting and congenial or marked by tension and pressure, and whether the work history indicates good adjustment. The pertinent factors in the past history will depend on the nature of the illnesses from which the patient has suffered.

No history of the patient's illness can be regarded as complete without at least brief inquiry into his personality structure. Illness invariably evokes in all patients some degree of anxiety that is responsible for the development of reactions that may often obscure the symptoms of the structural illness. These may in some instances become so pronounced as to dominate the picture. It is important to know therefore the manner of person who has developed the illness being probed. For this purpose a brief personality survey must be made, to include such diverse factors as the patient's relationship to other members of the family constellation, the educational and occupational histories, marital adjustment, and a brief personality sketch of the patient himself, covering his feelings, attitudes, goals, and frustrations.

Finally, information as to handedness should be sought, in an attempt to determine the laterality of cerebral dominance. This is of particular importance when one is dealing with patients suffering from disorders of language. The question as to which eye and which foot are predominant may need investigation, as well as family patterns of dexterity and dominance.

The main features of the history having been determined, the patient is then ready for examination.

THE NEUROLOGICAL EXAMINATION
CONSCIOUSNESS AND MENTATION

First, and most importantly, the state of awareness, i.e., consciousness and responsiveness, must be determined. If it is altered, the precise nature and degree of impairment should be defined (see Chapter 2). Particularly in the conscious and alert patient, of course, the physician is offered at the outset an opportunity to study various features of importance in the examination. The facial expression may be noted and impressions gained as to facial mobility and anxiety, as to whether the patient has a blank or rigid facies. The general intellectual level of the patient and his premorbid attainment may be roughly estimated by his vocabulary, the manner of presentation of the material having to do with his illness, by his occupation, and by his activities. Responses to questions concerning general fund of knowledge and culture also shed light on the intellectual background.

It should be possible by means of a bedside examination to determine whether there is evidence of intellectual impairment and whether there is clouding of the sensorium. If it is found that an intellectual deficit is in fact present, formal psychological testing may be of considerable value in measuring the extent of the deficit. It should be emphasized that decrease or loss of intellectual function is usually the result of structural brain disease; however, slowing of intellectual processes (bradyphrenia) may be found in depression and with severe anxiety or with other emotional disorders.

Early in the course of the examination, the patient's *orientation* for time, place, and person should be determined. *Memory,* both remote and recent, can be tested, often during the course of the history taking. Efforts should be made to determine dates of birth, marriage, graduation from school, and other pertinent data. Recent recall can be assessed by asking when and how the patient came to the hospital, by recalling the name of his physician, and his own address, and by determining his ability to give an adequate account of his own illness. He may be presented with simple stories and asked to repeat them and may be requested to memorize, and subsequently recall, the name of a flower, a hypothetical street address, etc. Test sentences, e.g., "There is one thing a nation needs to be strong and great and that is a firm, secure supply of wood," are sometimes used for this purpose as well. The *attention span,* vital to such tests of memory, is evaluated during the give-and-take of the history; it may more formally be investigated by tests of digit retention, with assessment of the ability to repeat series of digits forward and backward. When digits are presented at an even rate of one per second, the normal adult can recall and repeat approximately five or six forward, four or five in reverse. The *understanding* of simple and more complex commands can be determined during the course of the neurological examination and can be supplemented by asking the patient to perform acts of increasing complexity (put out your tongue; close your right eye, and raise your left hand, etc.). The fund of *general information* can be tested by inquiring the names of the President, the governor of the state, the capitals of states and countries, the dates of the principal wars, the names of rivers in the United States, and the like.

The ability to *calculate* should be tested routinely. The serial 7 test is most commonly employed for this purpose, the patient being requested to subtract 7 serially, beginning with 100; thus, $100 - 7$, $93 - 7$, etc. Other simple arithmetical problems can be tested (the number of inches in 3¾ feet; multiplication problems: if 5 times X equals 20, how much is X, etc.). In patients with limited educational background, calculations such as these may be a priori impossible, and more mundane arithmetical devices, such as a grocery shopping list, should be employed. The ability to think in the *abstract* must also be determined; this can be evaluated by asking the patient to explain common proverbs ("People who live in glass houses shouldn't throw stones," "A bird in the hand is worth two in the bush," "Don't cry over spilt milk," etc.), and to determine similarities in classes of objects ("Why is a cat like a lion?"). Again, those with an impoverished formal education and few day-to-day intellectual demands may think much more concretely than would ordinarily be anticipated. The *speech* can be examined during the course of the history taking, and it can be readily determined whether dysarthria or aphasia is present (see Chapter 2). In appropriate cases, specific language tests may be given. In patients with relatively mild disorders of expressive or receptive language or both, ordinary speech may not be grossly deranged, and correct identification of the defect may be possible only with such specific testing. Awareness of the relationships of one part of the body to another (*body scheme*), and of the body to extracorporeal space, must also be noted; when indicated, specific testing with drawings, such as of the face of a clock or a flower, with design copying and completion, and with construction of figures with matchsticks and varicolored cubes may be employed. Finally, efforts should be made through the history to determine impairment of *judgment* and *changes* in personality. The degree of insight into the illness can be assessed by inquiring whether the patient regards himself as being sick and requiring treatment. Abnormal trends such as delusions, hallucinations, obsessions, and phobias should be investigated in appropriate instances. The mood and general reaction of the patient to his illness can be determined by observation during the routine examination so that anxiety, depression, excitement, suspiciousness, and the like, may be readily determined.

THE CRANIAL NERVES

I. Olfactory

The olfactory nerve does not as a rule require detailed investigation for routine purposes; evaluation of its function is especially pertinent in instances of trauma, visual failure, and progressive intellectual deterioration. It is examined by closing one of the patient's nostrils and asking him to smell coffee or lemon extract with the other. A patent airway is essential for accurate testing. Tobacco, peppermint, vinegar, or other mildly aromatic substances may be used; highly volatile substances such as ammonia should be avoided. Distinction between odors is more important than precise identification of any given substance.

II. Optic

This is tested by direct examination of the optic nerve and by investigation of visual acuity and the visual fields. The optic nerve is examined by means of an ophthalmoscope. Every physician should learn its use, since information of great value in a variety of circumstances can be obtained from the fundus oculi. The visual acuity is tested by means of readily available standardized charts or, when such are not at hand, by determination of the ability to read various sizes of newsprint, counting fingers, etc. A description of the normal fundus can be found in any standard text of ophthalmology.

For accurate and complete study the visual fields must be examined by means of a perimeter and tangent screen. Gross visual field defects may be detected, however, by means of the confrontation test. This is performed by having the patient face the examiner at a distance of 2 or 3 feet, asking the patient to cover one eye with his hand and to fix his gaze on the examiner's nose. The examiner's finger is then brought in along the main axes of the visual field, nasal, temporal, superior, and inferior, the patient calling out as soon as the examiner's finger is seen. A corsage pin with a white head may be used for more accurate determinations; on occasion, colored objects, particularly red, prove useful. In instances of severe visual loss the fields may be mapped out by means of a flash-light. By means of the confrontation test gross hemianopic field defects may be disclosed. Scotomas may be detected also by this method; the patient's position in relation to the examiner remains as described, the patient being asked as the finger approaches to indicate where vision is lost in the visual field. With a cooperative patient, even the relative size of the blind spot can be determined at the bedside. When fields are tested by confrontation, stimuli should also be exposed simultaneously in both halves of the field; if this is not done, an attention visual defect may escape recognition. In stuporous patients, the response to a threatening stimulus on either side may be used as a crude guide to the integrity of the visual fields.

III, IV, VI. Ocular Nerves

All the ocular nerves are examined together.

PUPILLARY REFLEX. This is tested preferably in darkness, or shade, by flashing a light in the pupil and examining the size, regularity, shape, and reaction of the pupil. Normally the pupils are equal in size, regular in outline, and react promptly to direct light flashed into the eye. Under normal circumstances the pupil reacts quickly to light, the contraction being maintained for a very brief time and then relaxing as the sphincter of the iris fatigues with continued applica-

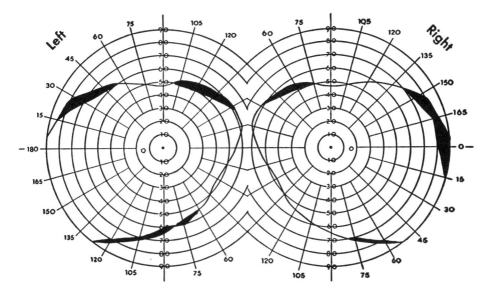

FIGURE 1-1. Normal visual fields showing the characteristic flattening above and on the nasal sides.

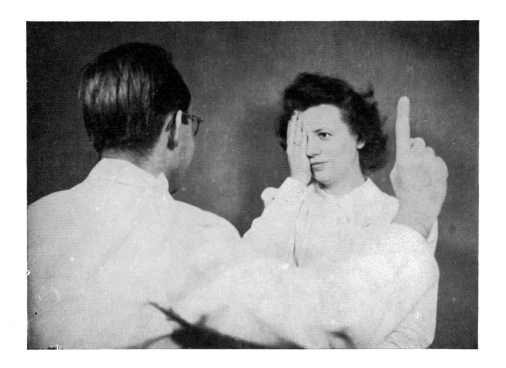

FIGURE 1-2. Confrontation method of determining the visual fields.

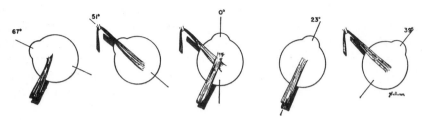

FIGURE 1-3.   Diagram illustrating the positions and actions of the vertical recti and oblique muscles in different positions of gaze of the right eye; the medial and lateral recti, which act solely as adductor or abductor of the globe respectively, are not indicated. (From Cogan, David: Neurology of the Ocular Muscles, ed. 2, 1963. Courtesy of Charles C Thomas, Publisher, Springfield, Ill.)

tion of the light.   A routine examination should include observation of the consensual response, the contraction of the pupil opposite to that directly stimulated by the light.   The accommodation reflex may be tested by watching the size of the pupil as it accommodates to near and far vision.

OCULAR MOVEMENTS.   Conjugate movements are tested by asking the patient to look to either side as far as he can or to follow a finger to either side as

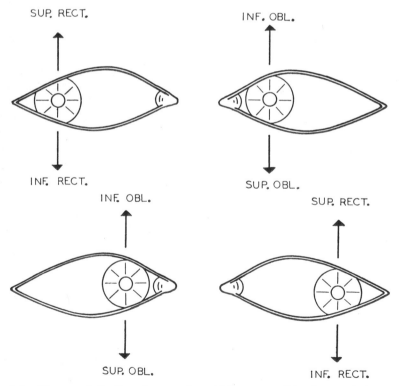

FIGURE 1-4.   Diagram indicating the muscles chiefly responsible for vertical movements of the eyes in different positions of gaze. (From Cogan, David: Neurology of the Ocular Muscles, ed. 2, 1963. Courtesy of Charles C Thomas, Publisher, Springfield, Ill.)

well as up and down. Individual eye muscle movements are tested by covering one eye and observing movement in all axes. Convergence is tested by asking the patient to look at the finger at a distance and on close examination. As the finger approaches the patient's nose the eyes are seen to converge inward and to maintain this converged position. Limitation of movement is looked for, and the patient is queried as to double vision. When a complaint of diplopia is elicited, one eye should be covered with a piece of red glass or plastic, and the patient asked to follow a moving light; this technique permits quick and accurate delineation of defective ocular movements by breaking up the images derived from the two eyes into differently colored and, thus, easily distinguished objects. The presence or absence of nystagmus is also noted.

V. Trigeminal

The *motor* portion of the nerve is tested by asking the patient to clench his teeth, the examiner feeling the masseter and temporal muscles in order to determine force of contraction and muscle bulk. The pterygoids may be tested by having the patient press the jaw laterally against the examiner's finger, the mouth being partially open. Deviation of the jaw due to masseter paralysis, or weakness, is determined by asking the patient to open the mouth, weakness being manifested by deviation of the jaw to the weak side. The *sensory* portion of the nerve is evaluated by testing the corneal reflex with a fine stimulator. The corneal reflex is extremely important under some circumstances, but as ordinarily elicited in routine fashion it has little value since in most instances it is brought out not by stimulation of the cornea but of the sclera. It must be tested in such a fashion that the testing stimuli is invisible to the patient since the latter will naturally blink on seeing an object approach the eye. For this purpose a fine hair mounted on an applicator, or a wisp of cotton, can be curved in such a way as to stimulate the cornea directly without being seen by the patient. The response consists of a rapid forceful contraction of the eyelid similar to that experienced when a foreign body enters the eye; a contralateral blink is common. When no response is obtained there is no contraction of the eyelid; this should always be checked by asking the patient whether the stimulus was felt. Facial sensation is examined by testing the skin of the face for touch, pain, and temperature sensations. The mucous membranes of the nose and mouth, and the anterior portion of the tongue, may also be tested.

VII. Facial

This nerve is examined by asking the patient to wrinkle the forehead, to frown (frontalis muscle), to close the eyelids tightly or to wink (orbicularis palpebrae muscle), to open the mouth, retract the mouth, blow out the cheeks, pucker the lips, screw up the nose, whistle, etc. (muscles of facial expression). By these various simple maneuvers the several muscles innervated by the facial nerve are tested and weakness or paralysis of the facial muscles easily detected. In addition to innervating the muscles of the face the facial nerve supplies taste innervation to the anterior two thirds of the tongue. This need not be tested routinely, but in cases of peripheral facial paralysis it becomes necessary to determine whether the taste fibers are involved. This is tested by having the patient protrude the tongue and applying at different times sugar, salt, and quinine. The patient is asked to detect the material used without pulling the tongue back into the mouth, an easy performance for the normal subject.

VIII. Auditory

Examination of the auditory nerve is carried out by testing the cochlear and the vestibular portions of the nerve.

COCHLEAR. This portion is concerned with hearing, which may be tested by observing the patient's ability to hear the spoken voice or a whisper. It may also be tested by simple tuning-fork procedures, using a C-512 or a higher pitched tuning fork. This is set in vibration, placed on the mastoid process, and the patient asked to let the examiner know when the vibration has ceased. At this point it is placed next to the ear and the patient asked whether the tuning fork is still heard. Under normal circumstances air conduction (AC) is greater than bone conduction (BC), and the fork will be heard here after it is no longer heard on the bone. Measurement may be made of the times over which the tuning fork is heard over the bone as compared with air, but for routine purposes this is not necessary. In nerve deafness, both air and bone conduction may be reduced, but the normal formula (AC > BC) pertains. On the other hand, in conduction deafness, bone conduction is better than air. Lateralization tests are also used. A tuning fork is placed on the forehead, and with one ear completely occluded by the examiner's finger, the patient is asked to tell on which side the vibration is loudest. Normally it is heard best on the occluded side. In conduction deafness the tuning fork is referred to the diseased ear, while in nerve deafness it is not heard on the affected side even with occlusion.

For more precise examination of audition, the audiometer is used. By means of this special instrument the degree of hearing loss and the frequencies in which it is affected may be accurately measured.

VESTIBULAR. This portion of the nerve is tested in a variety of ways. One such is the past-pointing test. The patient is asked to raise his arm and to bring the index finger down on the examiner's finger with the patient's arm outstretched, first with the eyes open, then with them closed. It is also carried out in the horizontal plane. Normally the patient's finger touches the examiner's without difficulty. In vestibular disease the finger past-points to one side or the other consistently. The function of the vestibular portion of the auditory nerve is also evaluated by a search for nystagmus (see Chapter 2). Briefly, this consists of a to-and-fro movement of the eyeballs, usually in the horizontal plane but sometimes in the vertical plane. It is examined by asking the patient to look to one side, the eyeballs moving to the extreme positions. True nystagmus is characterized by a sustained movement consisting of two components, a fast jerk to the side of the deviation and a slow jerk back to the midline. At times a rotary element is seen. Vertical nystagmus may be elicited on looking upward and, less commonly, downward; it consists of straight-up-and-down movements of the eyeballs in a vertical plane.

Special studies of vestibular function may also be performed. One such consists of stimulation of the semicircular canals by the injection of cold water (18° to 20° C.) slowly into the external auditory canal with the patient sitting upright. After the injection of 100 cc. of water or less, or after a blast of cold air, observations are made concerning the following features: (1) nystagmus, (2) past-pointing, (3) the occurrence of vertigo, nausea, or vomiting. With the patient in the upright position the vertical canals are stimulated; the responses of the horizontal canals may be tested by bending the patient's head forward. After irrigation of the ears normal responses of a definite sort are observed. Thus, after irrigation of the right ear one notes (1) vertigo within 2 minutes after irrigation is begun; (2) lateral and rotary nystagmus to the left; (3) past-pointing to the right; (4) nausea and sometimes vomiting; (5) increase of the nystagmus to the right side with the head flexed, and (6) intensification of the vertigo, nystagmus, and past-pointing on return of the head to the upright position. After irrigation of the left ear the subjective reactions such as nausea, vertigo, and vomiting remain the same, but nystagmus is to the right and past-pointing chiefly to the left.

[handwritten margin notes: CALORICS / FAST compunents COWS / PAST POINTING TO COLD S.05 / FALLING TO COLD S.05]

Under some circumstances, as in cerebellopontine angle tumor, no responses are obtained from the semicircular canals of one ear. In other cases the responses may be perverted, nystagmus occurring to the wrong side. In posterior fossa tumors the subjective responses such as nausea, vertigo, and vomiting may be completely absent or decreased; in tumors above the tentorium they may be greatly exaggerated.

It is often useful to observe the patient's ocular responses as a striped drum, or measuring tape, is moved before his eyes from one side to the other. This maneuver elicits a typical pattern of nystagmus referred to generally as opticokinetic nystagmus, which may be deranged in diseases of the posterior fossa as well as of the cerebral hemispheres.

IX. Glossopharyngeal

This nerve is tested routinely with the vagus nerve. Its chief function is sensory; it supplies the pharynx and posterior third of the tongue with taste fibers. Its only motor function has to do with movement of the pharynx by means of the stylopharyngeus muscle whose role in this function is so minor that it can hardly be tested.

X. Vagus

The vagus nerve has many functions. It is the chief motor nerve of the pharynx and larynx. It is tested routinely by observing pharyngeal movements. This is best done by asking the patient to phonate by saying "ah." Under normal circumstances the soft palate and uvula will be pulled up in the midline. In case of weakness of one side, the palate will be pulled up on phonation to the healthy side while the diseased side droops; in cases of bilateral paralysis there will be no palatal movement. The pharyngeal reflex may be tested by touching the back of the pharynx with a throat stick, with ensuing contraction of the palatal muscles under normal conditions.

The larynx may be tested by studying the timbre of the voice, the vocal musculature being supplied through the vagus by the recurrent laryngeal nerve. In case of hoarseness or aphonia, direct mirror laryngoscopy is advisable.

The vegetative functions of the vagus nerve such as pulse and respiration may also be tested.

XI. Spinal Accessory

This nerve innervates the trapezius and sternomastoid muscles. The function of the former is tested by asking the patient to shrug his shoulders against resistance and of the latter, by turning the head against resistance. Both sternomastoids may be tested simultaneously by having the patient flex his head forcefully against a resisting hand.

XII. Hypoglossal

This is the motor nerve of the tongue. It is tested by asking the patient to protrude the tongue. Under normal circumstances the tongue is protruded in the midline. In paralysis of the tongue, there is deviation to the paralyzed side. Power of the tongue may be tested by asking the patient to press the tongue against each cheek, the force of the protrusion being tested by the finger of the examiner pressing against the tongue. Atrophy and involuntary movements of the tongue are ordinarily apparent with simple inspection; evaluation of fibrillations requires that the tongue be at rest in the floor of the mouth.

For ordinary routine purposes in a busy general practice, examination of the visual fields, pupillary reflexes, ocular movements, facial innervation, and movements of the pharynx and tongue are most important, along with funduscopic observation. When possible, or when indicated by the patient's specific symptoms, a more complete examination is of course desirable.

MOTOR SYSTEM

Examination of the motor system includes the determination of muscle power, bulk, and tone, observation of the occurrence of involuntary muscle movements such as fasciculations and tremors, and assessment of the status of the reflexes. Evaluation of cerebellar function may also be considered within the general scope of this part of the examination.

For the determination of weakness or strength of the muscles a few simple maneuvers are sufficient; if more complex studies are necessary they may be carried out on the muscles indicated. Thus, fully detailed examination of the muscles of the shoulder and pelvic girdles is not routinely necessary, but in cases of shoulder or leg pain or weakness, careful evaluation of these muscles is essential.

Hands and Arms

The hand grips are tested by asking the patient to squeeze the examiner's fingers, it being first determined whether the patient is right- or left-handed. The power of the hand grip is determined by the force required to withdraw the fingers from the clenched fist. The patient is also asked to fix the tightly clenched fist at the wrist, the examiner attempting to overcome this maximum dorsiflexion. Abduction of the fingers against resistance, and opposition of the thumb, may also be tested simply and quickly. Power in the arms is tested by asking the patient to flex and extend the forearm against resistance. Abduction of the arms at the shoulders should also be tested. When there is a history of neck, shoulder, or arm pain, full examination of the shoulder girdle muscles is essential.

Legs and Feet

The legs are similarly tested by asking the patient to flex and extend them against resistance. Dorsiflexion of the feet is tested by asking the patient to push the partially flexed foot against the examiner's hand, and plantar flexion by pushing down against the examiner's hand; dorsiflexion and plantar flexion of the feet may also be tested by asking the patient to walk on the heels and toes. The power of extension of the leg at the knee and at the hip should also be evaluated.

While the musculature is being examined for signs of weakness, *muscle tone* should be investigated for changes such as flaccidity, spasticity, or rigidity. If a change of muscle tone is found, it should be determined whether this is focal or general.

Muscle atrophy should be searched for, and, if found, its distribution should be determined. Muscular fasciculations should always be sought, whether or not atrophy is present.

Involuntary movements such as chorea, athetosis, tics, or hemiballism should be noted.

To one who is well versed in the routine examination of the nervous system, all this and more can be performed very quickly and accurately in examination of the motor system. For ordinary routine purposes in which the neurological examination is part of a general physical survey of the patient, examination of the motor system may be confined to studying the power of the arms and legs, the state of the tendon reflexes, and the coordination of the limbs.

REFLEXES

Jaw Jerk

This is obtained by tapping the chin briskly when the mouth is held partially open; the normal response is closure of the jaw. Increased briskness of response is looked for. Not often tested, this reflex may be of substantial value in determining the segmental level of a lesion in patients exhibiting bilateral pyramidal tract signs.

Table 1-1. Important Deep Tendon Reflexes

	Elicited by	Response	Segmental Level
JAW	Tapping mandible in half-open position	Closure of jaw	Pons
SCAPULO-HUMERAL	Tapping vertebral border of scapula	Contraction of teres minor, infraspinatus, etc.	C5 and C6
TRICEPS	Tapping triceps tendon	Extension at elbow	C7 to D1
BICEPS	Tapping biceps tendon	Flexion at elbow	C5 and C6
RADIAL	Tapping styloid process of radius	Contraction of supinator longus	C5 and C6
KNEE	Tapping patellar tendon	Extension at knee	L3 and L4
ANKLE	Tapping Achilles tendon	Extension at ankle	S1 and S2

Biceps Reflex

This is examined by placing the elbow of the arm to be examined in the hand of the examiner, the examiner's thumb being placed over the biceps tendon and struck briskly with a reflex hammer. The result is flexion of the arm.

Brachioradial Reflex

This is elicited by tapping the lower third of the radius with the forearm midway between pronation and supination. The result is flexion of the forearm on the arm and, usually, also flexion of the fingers and hand. This is one of the most important reflexes of the arm but is often neglected. With a lesion in the fifth cervical segment, tapping of the radius causes flexion only of the hand and fingers but not of the forearm (inversion of the radial reflex). A similar response may be elicited in normal persons and has been found also in myopathies.

Triceps Reflex

This is tested by holding the arm of the patient supported under the elbow with the arm partly extended, the triceps tendon being tapped by the reflex hammer; extension of the arm results. In the supine position the arm is drawn across the chest, the forearm slightly flexed, and the triceps tendon tapped just above the olecranon.

Patellar Reflex

This is brought out by tapping the patellar tendon in the partly extended leg. If sought for with the patient in bed, placing a rolled pillow under the knees facilitates the reflex activity.

Achilles Reflex

The ideal method of eliciting this is with the patient lying on his face, the knee flexed, and the foot held slightly dorsiflexed by the examiner's hand; the Achilles tendon is struck in order to produce plantar flexion. It may also be tested by having the patient kneel on a chair while the Achilles tendon is struck, or by having the patient on his back with the legs flexed and everted, the Achilles tendon being struck while the foot is held dorsiflexed.

Plantar Reflex

For routine purposes the sole of the foot is stimulated by a blunt object carried along its outer side and thence across the ball of the foot. The normal response is flexion of the toes.

Abdominal Reflexes

These are elicited by running an object such as the blunt end of an orange stick, a pin, key, or brush along the upper and lower abdominal quadrants on either side. A normal response consists of movement of the abdominal musculature and a pull of the umbilicus toward the stimulated side. Maximal relaxation of the abdominal musculature is most favorable for the response; when the muscles have been unduly stretched, as by repeated pregnancies, the reflexes may be difficult or impossible to obtain.

Table 1-2. Important Superficial Reflexes

	Elicited by	*Response*	*Segmental Level*
CORNEAL	Touching cornea with hair	Contraction of orbicularis oculi	Pons
PHARYNGEAL	Touching posterior wall of pharynx	Contraction of pharynx	Medulla
PALATAL	Touching soft palate	Elevation of palate	Medulla
SCAPULAR	Stroking skin between scapulae	Contraction of scapular muscles	C5 to D1
EPIGASTRIC	Stroking downward from nipples	Dimpling of epigastrium ipsilaterally	D7 to D9
ABDOMINAL	Stroking beneath costal margins and above inguinal ligament	Contraction of abdominal muscles in quadrant stimulated	D8 to D12
CREMASTERIC	Stroking medial surface of upper thigh	Ipsilateral elevation of testicle	L1 and L2
GLUTEAL	Stroking skin of buttock	Contraction of glutei	L4 and L5
BULBO- CAVERNOUS	Pinching dorsum of glans	Contraction of bulbous urethra	S3 and S4
SUPERFICIAL ANAL	Pricking perineum	Contraction of rectal sphincters	S5 and coccygeal

Cremasteric Reflex

This is examined by stimulating the inner side of the thigh, the response being retraction of the testicle on that side.

When the tendon reflexes are difficult to obtain with ordinary techniques, the patient is asked to clench or squeeze his hands together while the examiner attempts to elicit the reflex. This maneuver, termed *reinforcement*, may bring out reflexes not otherwise obtainable.

Additional Reflexes

The *orbicularis oculi reflex* is elicited as follows: The skin at the outer corner of the eye is held between the thumb and index finger, pulling it back slightly, and the thumb is tapped lightly with a reflex hammer. There follows a reflex contraction of the orbicularis oculi muscle. Diminution of the reflex is found in facial palsies of peripheral origin. It is preserved in central facial palsies. The response obtained is a deep muscle reflex. The *scapulohumeral reflex* is elicited by tapping the vertebral border of the scapula with resulting contraction of muscles of the shoulder girdle and arm. Many muscles are brought into play, especially the deltoid, pectoralis major, infraspinatus, and teres minor. Abduction of the arm occurs. Unilateral absence of the reflex is found in lesions of the fifth cervical segment. The *adductor reflex of the thigh* is obtained by placing the finger on the medial condyle of the femur with the leg slightly abducted. When the finger is tapped, adduction of the leg follows. The *biceps femoris reflex* is best elicited with the patient lying on the side opposite the one being examined, the leg being bent at the hip and knee. The finger is placed on the hamstring tendon and is tapped with a reflex hammer. Contraction of the muscle results. The *pharyngeal reflex* is elicited by touching the posterior wall of the pharynx, contraction of the pharynx resulting. The *scapular reflex*, elicited by stroking the skin between the scapulae, results in contraction of the scapular muscles. The *gluteal reflex* results in contraction of the glutei on stroking the skin of the buttock.

CEREBELLAR SYSTEM

A survery should routinely be made of the cerebellar system, the function of which is to coordinate movements into smooth and effectual patterns. Tests are directed both to the limbs and to the trunk.

Arms

Finger-Nose Test

The patient is asked to place the index finger of either hand on the nose. This is normally performed smoothly and easily with eyes both open and closed. This test may be varied by asking the patient to touch the nose in rapid succession several times.

Finger-Finger Test

The patient is asked to place the index finger of his hand on the examiner's index finger. This may be repeated several times in rapid succession.

Pronation-Supination Test

With the arms extended in front of him the patient is asked to pronate and supinate rapidly, using the elbows as a fulcrum. Under normal circumstances the movements are of equal amplitude, smooth and even, and there is no tendency on the part of the arms to drift outward or inward during the movement. The beat and rhythm are well maintained.

Patting Test

The patient is requested to pat rapidly the examiner's hand or his own leg. Under normal conditions this is performed with even amplitude and a smooth rhythm.

Rebound Test

The ability to check movements quickly, with coordinated action of agonists, antagonists, and synergists, is tested by observing the response to sudden passive displacement of the outstretched arms. Normally such a movement is rapidly checked, the displaced limb returning to its former position smoothly and accurately.

Legs

Heel-Knee Test

With the patient in the supine position the heel of one foot is placed on the opposite knee. This is done smoothly, without tremor and with accuracy. The foot may then be slid down the shin, again a movement normally performed smoothly and evenly.

Patting Test

The patient is asked to pat his foot quickly on the floor, the test being similar to this performed in the arms.

Figure-of-Eight-Test

While recumbent, the patient draws a figure-of-eight in the air with his great toe. This is ordinarily performed smoothly and with dispatch.

Trunk

Gait

Testing the gait constitutes a good method of determining truncal coordination. In order to do this the patient should be given plenty of room and asked to walk briskly with the eyes open and closed and to turn quickly. He should also be requested to walk heel-to-toe in a straight line (tandem gait); this can be done normally without loss of balance.

He may also be asked to walk around a chair and to sit and rise quickly from a chair, in order to test the ability to make rapid postural adjustments. The patient may be asked also to arise from a reclining posture without a pillow and with the legs widely separated.

The station is tested routinely, the patient being asked to stand in Romberg's position with the feet close together, first with the eyes open, then with the eyes closed. He is additionally asked to stand with one foot directly in front of the other (tandem Romberg).

For ordinary purposes the finger-nose, heel-knee, and pronation-supination tests, as well as evaluation of the gait and station, will suffice to determine cerebellar function.

SENSORY SYSTEM

A complete sensory examination includes the investigation of touch, pain, heat, cold, position, and vibration senses, as well as of a variety of discriminatory modalities. For an accurate sensory examination the patient should be examined in a quiet room where he is not distracted by extraneous stimuli and preferably when he is not fatigued. The examination should not be too lengthy, since fatigue sets in rapidly and the replies become increasingly inaccurate. In routine examinations, sensation is usually tested at the end of the examination. If sensory changes are found this part of the examination should be repeated alone.

Examination of sensation consists of three portions. (1) Qualitative, to determine what elements of sensation are affected. (2) Quantitative, to determine the degree of involvement of sensation when it is impaired. (3) Regional, to map out the areas of sensory impairment or loss. In the normal subject only the qualitative aspects of sensation are studied, it being determined that sensation is well appreciated over the body surface and equally felt over both sides of the body, limbs, and face. In cases of sensory impairment, it becomes necessary to investigate the degree of sensory loss and the distribution of this loss. Complete sensory loss is spoken of as anesthesia (touch), analgesia (pain), etc.; partial sensory loss is referred to as hypalgesia, etc. In some instances, sensation is more keenly felt than normal; this is referred to as hyperesthesia, hyperalgesia, etc. It is extremely important in every case of sensory loss to determine the exact distribution of the loss in order to determine whether it corresponds with peripheral nerve or with root distribution, whether it is a complete sensory level as seen in transverse spinal cord lesions, or hemianesthesia, or a dissociated sensory syndrome (see Chapter 3).

Touch

This sense is tested by means of a cotton wisp or by a camel's-hair brush, or even by the examiner's finger, which is brought gingerly and lightly down on the skin. Tickling should be avoided, since this modality may actually represent subliminal pain.

Pain

Pain is tested by means of a pin with which the patient is pricked over various parts of the skin's surface. The qualitative aspect is examined by determining whether the patient appreciates correctly the pin prick over various parts of the body, the patient being asked to distinguish between the point and the head of the pin. Examination for "extinction" or "inattention" is often important in determining sensory defects. This is tested by simultaneously stimulating opposite sides of the body symmetrically and determining whether pin prick is obliterated on one side while still appreciated on the other.

Heat and Cold

They are tested by utilizing test tubes containing hot water and cracked ice. These are extremes of temperature that suffice for routine neurological examination. The patient, with the eyes closed, is asked to identify heat and cold over various parts of the body.

Vibration Sense

This is examined by means of a C-128 tuning fork applied over the elbow, wrist, ankle, and shin. The tuning fork is set in active vibration, and the patient, with the eyes closed, is asked to identify the sensation. He is also asked to determine when the vibration ceases, the examiner interrupting the vibration as he desires. In doubtful instances a crude quantitative test may be made, the patient being asked to determine how long he feels the vibration over the back of the hand or tibia. Rough clinical tests with a C-128 tuning fork indicate that vibration is felt over the back of the hand for an average of 15 to 20 seconds, and over the tibia for 7 to 10 seconds in young subjects. In patients over 50 years of age, vibration sense is often impaired in the legs.

Position Sense

This modality is examined by grasping the sides of the thumb or great toe and gently moving it, the patient being asked to determine whether the digit is pointing up or down. Recognition of the initiation of movement may also be sought.

Special Sensory Examinations

Two-point discrimination is examined by means of a calibrated compass. The patient is asked to indicate whether he feels one or two compass points over various parts of the body. The test is important in diseases of the sensory cortex and in peripheral nerve disease. The threshold, or minimal recognizable separation, is 4 or 5 mm. in the finger tips, but much greater elsewhere. *Tactile localization* is tested with the patient's eyes closed, by touching a spot on the skin, the patient being asked to indicate the spot touched by placing his finger on it. Normally localization is quite accurate over the fingers and hands, relatively less precise more proximally.

Graphesthesia consists of the ability to recognize numbers or letters traced on the skin with a blunt object. The patient is asked to identify the number or letter so drawn.

Stereognosis is tested by asking the patient, with the eyes closed, to identify the size and shape of an object placed in the hand.

Differences in texture and weight may be tested by asking the patient to identify various textures of cloth and to determine the difference in the weight of standardized blocks.

Table 1-3.   Muscle Innervation

(*After Raezer*)

ORDER OF ARRANGEMENT: *Muscle action; muscles with spinal cord segments* (C—cervical, T—thoracic, L—lumbar, S—sacral); *cord of plexus—peripheral nerve.* Asterisks (*) indicate the muscles chiefly responsible for the movement in question.

UPPER EXTREMITY—BRACHIAL PLEXUS—C5 to T1

1. FLEXORS AND LATERAL ROTATORS OF HEAD:
   *a. Sternocleidomastoid m.—medulla and C2, C3, C4—Cranial Nerve XI
   b. Posterior neck m.—C2, C3, C4 and nerves
      i   Longus capitis
      ii Rectus capitis anterior
      iii Longus colli

2. EXTENSORS OF HEAD:
   a. Trapezius m.—medulla and C2, C3, C4—Cranial Nerve XI
   b. Posterior neck m.—C2, C3, C4 and nerves
      *i Longissimus capitis
      ii Semispinalis capitis

3. ELEVATORS OF SHOULDERS: Test: Shrugging of shoulders
   *a. Trapezius m.—same as 2a
   b. Elevators of scapula—C3, C4, C5—dorsal scapular n.
      i   Levator scapulae
      ii Rhomboidei

Table 1-3—Continued

4. RETRACTORS OF SHOULDERS:
    *a. Trapezius m.—same as 2 a
    b. Rhomboidei—same as 3b

5. LATERAL ABDUCTORS OF ARM: *Above 90° angle* (also fix scapula below 90°)
    a. Trapezius m.—same as 2a
    b. Anterior serratus m.—C5, C6, C7—long thoracic n.

6. FORWARD THRUSTING OF ARM: Test: Patient extends arms forward placing the palms against a wall and pushes body toward the wall keeping the arms extended. Examiner observes scapula for "winging" (separation of scapula from back) with the inferior angle of the scapula pulled up and in
    a. Anterior serratus m.—same as 5b

7. ADDUCTORS OF HUMERUS:
    *a. Latissimus dorsi m.—C6, C7, C8—posterior cord of brachial plexus—thoracodorsal n.
    *b. Pectoralis major m.—C5 to T1—lateral and medial cords—anterior thoracic n.
    c. Teres major m.—C5, C6—posterior cord—subscapularis n.
    d. Teres minor m.—C5, C6—posterior cord—axillary n.
    e. Coracobrachialis m.—C5, C6—musculocutaneous n.

8. FLEXORS OF HUMERUS: Test: Arm at side pushing forward against resistance—"punching" action
    *a. Pectoralis major and minor m.—same as 7b
    b. Deltoid m.—C5, C6—axillary n.
    c. Subscapularis m.—C5, C6—posterior cord—subscapularis n.
    d. Coracobrachialis m.—same as 7e

9. EXTENSORS OR RETRACTORS OF ARM: *Test*: Arm and elbow at side pushing back against resistance—"swimming" action
    *a. Latissimus dorsi m.—same as 7a

10. ABDUCTORS OF ARM: Test: Arm laterally abducted *up to 90° angle*
    a. Initiator of abduction—C5, C6—suprascapular n.
        i Supraspinatus m.
    *b. Deltoid m.—same as 8b.

11. MUSCLES OF RESPIRATION:
    a. *Normal respiration:*
        i Diaphragm—C3, C4, C5—phrenic n.
        ii Intercostals
        iii Subcostals   } T1 to T12—intercostal n
        iv Levator costarum
        v Scaleni—C4, C5—cervical nerves
    b. *Accessory muscles of respiration:*
        i Sternocleidomastoid m.—same as 1a
        ii Trapezius m.—same as 2a
        iii Anterior serratus m.—same as 5b
        iv Latissimus dorsi m. (coughing)—same as 7a
        v Pectoralis major and minor—same as 7b
        vi Rhomboidei m.—same as 3b
        vii Supraspinatus m.—same as 10a

Table 1-3—Continued

12. MEDIAL OR INWARD ROTATORS OF ARM: Test: Arm extended at side and rotated inward against resistance:
  a. Pectoralis major m.—same as 7b
  b. Latissimus dorsi m.—same as 7a
  c. Teres major m.—same as 7c
  d. Subscapularis m.—same as 8c
  e. Deltoid m.—same as 8b

13. LATERAL OR OUTWARD ROTATORS OF ARM: Test: Arm held at side and laterally rotated against resistance:
  a. Teres minor m.—same as 7d
  b. Infraspinatus m.—same as 10a
  c. Deltoid m.—same as 8b

14. FLEXORS OF FOREARM (elbow):
  a. *Chief flexors:* C5, C6—lateral cord—musculocutaneous n.
    *i Biceps brachii
    ii Brachialis
    iii Coracobrachialis
  b. *Accessory flexors:*
    i   Brachioradialis—C5, C6—posterior cord—radial n.
    ii Pronator teres—C6—median n.
    iii Palmaris longus—C6—median n.

15. EXTENSORS OF FOREARM (elbow):
  a. Triceps brachii m.—C6, C7, C8—posterior cord—radial n.
  b. Anconeus—same as triceps

16. PRONATORS OF FOREARM (rotation of forearm inward):
  a. Pronator teres—C6—median n.
  b. Pronator quadratus—C7, C8—median n.
  c. Flexor carpi radialis—same as pronator teres

17. SUPINATORS OF FOREARM (rotation of forearm outward):
  a. *Supinator m.:* C5, C6—posterior cord—radial n.
     (arm extended)
  b. *Biceps brachii:* Same as 4a
     (arm flexed)

18. FLEXORS OF WRIST:
  a. *Main flexors:* C6—median n.
    i   Flexor carpi radialis
    ii Palmaris longus
    iii Flexor digitorum sublimis
  b. *Accessory flexion:*
    i   Flexor carpi ulnaris—C8, T1—ulnar n.
    ii Flexor digitorum profundus—C6, T1—median and ulnar nerves

19. EXTENSORS OF WRIST: All innervated by C6, C7, C8—radial n.
  a. Extensor carpi radialis longus }
  b. Extensor carpi radialis brevis } extend wrist

Table 1-3—Continued

  c. Extensor digitorum communis—extends all phalanges of fingers
  d. Extensor digiti quinti proprius—extends phalanges of little finger
  e. Extensor carpi ulnaris—extends ulnar side of wrist
  f. Extensor pollicis brevis—extends proximal phalanx of thumb
  g. Extensor pollicis longus—extends distal phalanx of thumb
  h. Extensor indicis proprius—extends index finger

20. ADDUCTORS OF WRIST: Movement of wrist toward the ulna
  a. Flexor carpi ulnaris—same as 18b
  b. Extensor carpi ulnaris—same as 19e

21. ABDUCTORS OF WRIST:
  a. Flexor carpi radialis: Same as 18a
  b. Extensors that abduct: Same as 19
     i Extensor carpi radialis longus and brevis
     ii Extensor pollicis longus and brevis
  c. Abductor pollicis longus (abductor of base of thumb):
     C6, C7, C8—radial n.

HAND

I. MOVEMENTS OF THUMB:
  1. *Abduction of thumb:*
    a. Abductor pollicis brevis (abducts first metacarpal)—C6, C7—median n.
    b. Abductor pollicis longus—C6, C7, C8—radial n.
  2. *Extensors of thumb:* C6, C7, C8—radial n.
    a. Extensor pollicis longus and brevis
  3. *Adductor of thumb:* (pure adduction of thumb when thumb is on a plane with the hand)
    a. Adductor pollicis—C8, T1—ulnar n.
  4. *Flexor of thumb:* C6, C7—median n.
    a. Proximal phalanx—flexor pollicis brevis
    b. Terminal phalanx—flexor pollicis longus
  5. *Opposition of thumb to fingers:* C6, C7—median n.
    a. Opponens pollicis—assisted by
      i Flexor pollicis brevis—4a
      ii Adductor pollicis—3

II. MOVEMENTS OF SMALL FINGER: C8, T1—ulnar n.
  1. *Abductor of little finger:*
    a. Abductor digiti quinti
  2. *Flexor of little finger:*
    a. Flexor digiti quinti
  3. *Opposition of little finger to thumb:*
    a. Opponens digiti quinti
  N.B. All 3 of the above muscles act only on the metacarpophalangeal joint

III. MOVEMENTS OF FINGERS:
  1. *Flexor of metacarpophalangeal joints:* C6—median n.
    a. Flexor digitorum sublimis

Table 1-3—Continued

2. *Flexor of distal interphalangeal joints:* C7 to T1—median and ulnar n.
   a. Flexor digitorum profundus
3. *Extensor of all joints of 4 fingers:* C6, C7, C8—radial n.
   a. Extensor digitorum profundus
   b. Extensor digiti quinti proprius
   c. Extensor indicis proprius
4. *Accessory extensors of interphalangeal joints and flexors of metacarpophalangeal joints*
   a. Lateral 2 lumbricales—C7 to T1—median n.
   b. Medial 2 lumbricales—C8, T1—ulnar n.
   c. Interossei m.—C8, T1—ulnar n.
5. *Ab*ductors (spreading) and *ad*ductors (approximating) of fingers—C8, T1—ulnar n.
   a. Interossei m.
      i 4 volar interossei *ad*duct
      ii 4 dorsal interossei *ab*duct
6. *Thenar eminence of hand:* Muscles at base of thumb—C6, C7, C8, T1
7. *Hypothenar eminence of hand:* Muscles at base of little finger—C8, T1

SUMMARY OF MUSCLE INNERVATION
UPPER EXTREMITY

1. All movements of head and neck are initiated through the medulla and C2, C3, and C4—cranial nerve XI and respective cervical nerves.

2. Shrugging and retraction of shoulders mediated through the medulla and C2, C3, C4, and C5—cranial nerve XI and respective cervical nerves.

3. Paralysis of deltoid alone with normal flexion of wrist and metacarpophalangeal joints localizes the lesion to C5 segment.

4. Abduction and lateral rotation of arm, flexion of the elbow and supination of the forearm are all carried out through C5 and C6 segments *only*.

5. Flexion of metacarpophalangeal joints of the 4 fingers is mediated only by C6 segment.

6. Retraction of arm (swimming action) is initiated through C6, C7, and C8—thoracodorsal nerve.

7. Retraction of the arm, extension of the elbow, wrist and all the fingers, abduction of the wrist and thumb, and pronation of the forearm are all mediated through C6, C7, and C8 segments.

8. Flexion of the terminal phalanges of all 5 fingers is initiated through C7, C8, and T1 segments.

9. The muscles of the hypothenar eminence of the hand and interossei are innervated by C8 and T1 only through the ulnar nerve.

10. Adduction, flexion, and medial rotation of humerus initiated through C5 to T1 and all portions of the brachial plexus.

The ten summary movements noted above will be seen to follow a natural progression of movement. This will be made more clear if one performs these movements for himself in the order in which they are written. Furthermore this will aid greatly in fixing the above pattern and make memorization less arduous.

It should be noted that No. 10 is a set of movements that include the whole brachial plexus and hence are always involved to a greater or lesser extent with any lesion of the brachial plexus, or cord segments from C5 to T1.

Table 1-3—Continued

LOWER EXTREMITY

LUMBOSACRAL PLEXUS—L1 to S2

1. FLEXORS OF HIP JOINT: L2, L3 and L4
   *a. Iliopsoas m.—L2, L3 and L4—ant. rami of L2, L3 and L4 and femoral n.
   b. Rectus femoris ⎫
   c. Pectineus m. ⎬ L2, L3 and L4—femoral n.
   d. Sartorius m. ⎭
   e. *Ad*ductor longus and brevis ⎫
   f. *Ab*ductor magnus ⎬ L3 and L4—obturator n.
   g. Obturator externus ⎭

2. ADDUCTORS OF THIGH: L2, L3 and L4
   a. Adductor magnus ⎫
      i Adductor longus ⎪
      ii Adductor brevis ⎬ L2, L3 and L4—obturator n.
   b. Gracilis ⎪
   c. Obturator externus ⎭
   d. Sartorius m. ⎫ L2, L3—femoral n.
   e. Pectineus m. ⎭

3. EXTENSION OF KNEE: L3, L4 (±L5, S1)
   *a. Quadriceps femoris—L3, L4
   b. Tensor fasciae latae—L4 (L5 and S1)—superior gluteal n.

4. ABDUCTORS OF FEMUR: L4, L5, S1 (S2)
   a. Gluteus medius ⎫
   b. Gluteus minimus ⎬ L4, L5, S1—superior gluteal n.
   c. Tensor fasciae latae ⎭
   d. Superior and inferior gemelli m. ⎫
   e. Obturator internus m. ⎬ S1, S2—anterior rami n.
   f. Piriformis m. ⎭

5. EXTENSORS OF HIP:
   a. Gluteus maximus—L5, S1, S2—inferior gluteal n.
   b. Biceps femoris m. ⎫
   c. Semitendinosus m. ⎬ L5, S1, S2—sciatic n.
   d. Semimembranosus m. ⎭

6. LATERAL ROTATORS OF THIGH: L2 to S2
   a. Sartorius—same as 2d
   b. Adductor magnus, longus and brevis—same as 2a
   c. Obturator externus—same as 2c
   d. Gluteus maximus—same as 5a
   e. Biceps femoris (when knee is flexed)—same as 5b
   f. Inferior gemellus m.—same as 4d
   g. Piriformis m.—same as 4f
   h. Obturator internus m.—same as 4e
   i. Superior gemellus m.—same as 4d

Table 1-3—Continued

7. MEDIAL ROTATORS OF FEMUR: L4, L5, S1
    a. Tensor fasciae latae—same as 3b
    b. Gluteus medius and minimus—same as 4a and 4b
    c. Adductor magnus m.—same as 2a

8. FLEXORS OF KNEE: L2 to S2
    a. Sartorius—same as 2d
    b. Gracilis—same as 2b
    c. Biceps femoris—same as 5b
    d. Semitendinosus ⎫
    e. Semimembranosus ⎬ same as 5c and 5d
    f. Gastrocnemius—S1, S2—tibial n.

9. DORSIFLEXORS OF ANKLE (foot): L4, L5, S1—deep peroneal n.
    a. Tibialis anticus m.
    b. Extensor digitorum longus m.
    c. Peroneus tertius
    d. Extensor hallucis longus

10. EXTENSORS OF TOES: L4, L5 and S1—deep peroneal n.
    a. Extensor digitorum longus and brevis
    b. Extensor hallucis longus

11. PLANTAR FLEXORS OF FOOT: L4, L5, S1, S2
    a. Peroneus longus and brevis—L4, L5, S1—superficial peroneal n.
    b. Gastrocnemius m.—S1, S2—tibial n.
    c. Soleus
    d. Flexor digitorum longus ⎫
    e. Flexor hallucis longus ⎬ L5, S1, S2—tibial n.
    f. Tibialis posticus

12. INVERSION OF FOOT: L4, L5, S1
    a. Tibialis anticus—L4, L5, S1—deep peroneal n.
    b. Tibialis posticus—L5, S1—tibial n.

13. EVERSION OF FOOT: L4, L5, S1
    a. Peroneus tertius—L4, L5, S1—*deep* peroneal n.
    b. Peroneus longus and brevis—L4, L5, S1—*superficial* peroneal n.

14. MEDIAL ROTATORS OF FOOT (with knee flexed and foot flat on floor): L4 to S2
    a. Semitendinosus ⎫
    b. Semimembranosus ⎬ same as 5c and 5d
    c. Sartorius m. ⎫
    d. Gracilis m. ⎬ same as 2b and 2d
    e. Popliteus m.—L4, L5, S1—tibial n.

15. LATERAL ROTATOR OF FOOT WITH KNEE FLEXED:
    a. Bicep femoris m.—L5, S1, S2—sciatic n.

Table 1-3—Continued

16. PLANTAR FLEXORS OF TOES: L4 to S2
    a. Flexor digitorum longus
    b. Lumbricales (same action as in hand) } L5 to S2—tibial n.
    c. Flexor hallucis longus
    d. *Ab*ductor hallucis longus
    e. Flexor digitorum brevis } L4, L5, S1—medial plantar n.—branch of tibial n.
    f. Flexor hallucis brevis
    g. Flexor digiti quinti brevis
    h. Interossei } S1, S2—lateral plantar n.—branch of tibial n.
    i. Quadratus plantae m.

17. EXTERNAL ANAL SPHINCTER: S3, S4—pudendal n.

SUMMARY OF MUSCLE INNERVATION

LOWER EXTREMITY

1. Flexion of hip, sitting up, and adduction of femur mediated by L2, L3, and L4

2. Extension of knee mediated by L3 and L4 (exception—tensor fasciae latae—L4 to S1)

3. Therefore—dissociation in strength between flexion of the hip and adduction of the thigh on the one hand and extension of the knee on the other points to an exquisite lesion of L2 or L4 (sartorius muscle will be weak if such is the case).

4. Abduction and medial rotation of femur, dorsiflexion of foot, extension of toes, inversion and eversion of foot are all innervated by L4, L5, and S1.

5. If patient can adduct (L2, L3, and L4) the femur, and has poor abduction of the femur—a lesion of L5 and S1 is indicated.

6. Poor abduction of femur associated with normal strength in the gastrocnemius, soleus, and muscles of lateral half of foot isolates the lesion to L5.

7. Atrophy of muscles on the lateral half of the sole of the foot with some atrophy and weakness of the calf muscles (gastrocnemius and soleus muscle) and good flexion of *all* the toes—the lesion may be postulated to involve S1 and S2 with sparing of L5.

8. Ability to walk on heels reflects integrity of L4, L5, and S1.

9. Ability to walk on toes reflects integrity of L5, S1, and S2.

10. Injury to common peroneal nerve (especially over head of fibula) results in loss of dorsiflexion and loss of ability to evert the foot—foot is inverted with plantar flexion.

11. Injury to the deep peroneal nerve produces weakness or paralysis of dorsiflexion of foot with ability to evert the foot intact.

12. Injury to superficial peroneal nerve leaves dorsiflexion of foot intact and produces weakness or paralysis of eversion of the foot.

Generally: The anterior thigh muscles represent the upper lumbar cord segments and nerves; anterolateral aspect of the lower leg, the lower lumbar cord segments; the posterior thigh and leg, the lower lumbar and upper sacral cord segments; and the sole, the upper sacral cord segments. The external anal sphincter tone is supplied by the third and fourth sacral cord segments.

BIBLIOGRAPHY

Cogan, D. G.: Neurology of the Ocular Muscles, ed. 2. Charles C Thomas, Springfield, Ill., 1963.

DeJong, ĸ.: The Neurological Examination. Paul B. Hoeber, New York, 1967.

Denny-Brown, D. E.: Handbook of Neurological Examination and Case Recording, Rev. Ed. Harvard University Press, Cambridge, Mass., 1957.

McDowell, F., and Wolff, H. G.: Handbook of Neurological Diagnostic Methods. Williams and Wilkins Co., Baltimore, 1960.

Medical Research Council, War Memorandum No. 7 (rev. 2nd ed., 1943): Aids to the Investigation of Peripheral Nerve Injuries. Her Majesty's Stationery Office, London, reprinted 1967.

CHAPTER 2

Interpretation
of Neurological Symptoms
and Signs

An exhaustive survey of the meaning of neurological symptoms and signs would lead too far afield, yet some consideration of this aspect of the neurological examination is essential for the reason that the attainment of a logical diagnosis begins with recognition of abnormal signs, followed by their proper analysis and their grouping into a proper diagnosis. The chief abnormal findings that may be encountered in a neurological examination therefore merit some description.

CONSCIOUSNESS AND MENTATION

When a patient exhibits alterations in the state of awareness an effort should be made to grade the changes in terms of severity or depth; this may be of considerable importance in judging the course of the patient's illness, and, thus, of substantial import prognostically. *Lethargy* indicates a state of drowsiness or inattention, the patient dropping off to sleep frequently although rousable to command. Responses may be delayed or incomplete, and little spontaneity is seen. In *stupor* the degree of physical and mental activity is minimal; the patient can be roused only with difficulty, and responds inadequately to events about him. Primitive reflexes such as the suck or snout may appear. A loss of the ability to respond

33

to verbal stimuli with preservation of at least some arousal with painful stimuli is found in *semicoma*. Here, a decrease in the tendon reflexes may be encountered, and the plantar reflexes are often extensor. Eye movements may be wandering or dysconjugate. In *coma* there is no consistent response to either auditory or painful stimuli except perhaps for decerebrate or decorticate posturing. Reflexes are lost, periodic or depressed respirations are common, and pupillary abnormalities are frequent. The term *coma vigil*, or *akinetic mutism*, refers to a state of unresponsiveness in which the patient may open the eyes and appear aware, but in which he exhibits neither vocal nor motor responses except for occasional primitive manifestations such as sucking or swallowing.

Confusion is a state characterized by an inability to think with ordinary clarity and coherence, usually associated with a lack of spontaneous speech and often observed in lethargic individuals. Perceptual misinterpretations and distortions are common. Disorientation, particularly as to time and date, is frequently found. When psychomotor and autonomic overactivity are added to the syndrome of confusion the term *delirium* is employed; a *beclouded delirium* is a delirious state added to an antecedent dementia.

Many disorders, both focal and generalized, may be associated with the appearance of these states of altered awareness and response; these will be discussed in Chapter 3.

In testing of *mentation*, the responses of the patient must be analyzed carefully. Slow, hesitant replies are of great significance, provided it can be determined that they are not normal for the individual in question. Such slowness, which may be looked upon as an expression of delay in the processing of symbolic bits of information, is commonly observed in the individual with organic intellectual impairment but may also be found in the patient with aphasia. The *organic mental syndrome* appears in a number of circumstances and is characterized by loss or impairment of memory, especially for recent events, difficulty in concentration, impairment of ability to comprehend abstract concepts and to synthesize ideas, impairment of learning capacity, difficulty with simple arithmetical problems. Changes in personality and mood often appear. It may appear in any condition that causes diffuse or extensive destruction of the cerebral cortex or underlying white matter. The term *dementia* is often used interchangeably with *organic mental syndrome*, and diseases so characterized are commonly called *dementing* in nature.

The personality changes found in organic brain disease are not specifically indicative of frontal lobe disease, as is often thought, but do occur with disorders of these areas particularly frequently. The fundamental feature is a change in the normal mode of reaction of the affected person. Mistakes in judgment, loss of niceties of social behavior, coarse behavior, sexual excesses and indiscretions, and many other nonspecific forms of reaction are encountered. The type of reaction varies widely for each patient, but the important fact is, that, as compared with the premorbid personality, there is a change in the reactions of the patient. Mood disturbances, and in particular rapid mood swings, occur with organic brain disease. They have no localizing significance and are usually associated with diffuse lesions. Emotional lability may be seen in multiple sclerosis, or in senile or presenile dementias, and is characterized by loss of control and easy crying and laughing without adequate stimulus. Impulsive behavior is found at times in postencephalitic states and in epilepsy. Apathy may develop in the course of many organic disorders. Euphoria is common in multiple sclerosis; it may reflect a lack of insight as a result of loss of the patient's ability to assess and evaluate his own deficit. A curious syndrome of facetiousness with senseless jokes and puns may also be encountered in individuals with disease of the cerebrum and is referred to as *witzelsucht*. Depression may occur with intrinsic brain disease but often is reactive in nature.

Among the higher skilled or integrative acts that may be disturbed in patients with organic disease of the brain is language. This may be manifested by aphasia, i.e., disorder of symbolic language, or by dysarthria, which refers merely to disturbance in enunciation. *Aphasia* (see Chapter 3), or dysphasia, is characterized by a difficulty in the expression or comprehension of language. It may be evidenced simply by a readily identifiable inability to find words, a defect of which the patient is ordinarily aware and capable of describing, or by a severe and disabling defect in expression, with considerable loss of words, or in a gross defect in understanding, or in a combination of these. Minor deficits may be missed unless careful testing is pursued. Other defects in symbolic language, i.e., an inability to read (dyslexia, alexia) and to write (dysgraphia, agraphia), commonly accompany the disorder of spoken language. The term *dysarthria,* on the other hand, refers to impairment in the rate, rhythm, quality, and intonation of the voice and in the modulation (prosody) and articulation of sounds. Dysarthria is due to a defect in the muscular control of the peripheral speech apparatus, the central symbolic aspect of language being preserved. It is often tested by requesting the patient to repeat certain test phrases, such as "Massachusetts artillery," "particular statistics," "truly rural," "Irish constabulary," and "round the rugged rock the ragged rascal ran." Dysarthria may be due to lesions of either the central or the peripheral nervous system. Various forms can be identified whose recognition may yield important information as to location and nature of the underlying disease process. For example, in instances of pseudobulbar palsy a *spastic dysarthria* is encountered, characterized by imprecision of consonants, monotony of pitch, and irregular loudness, along with a strained almost strangled quality. The voice may be nasal. Nasality is much more prominent in the *flaccid dysarthria* of bulbar palsy and is looked upon as due to weakness of the palatal, pharyngeal, and lingual muscles. The speech is quite muffled, often with a slow and sibilant quality, and defective articulation of consonants is found. In amyotrophic lateral sclerosis, features of both bulbar and pseudobulbar speech are identifiable; inappropriate silences and gaps between words and prolongation of phonemes are additionally encountered. The dysarthria of cerebellar disease is considered a reflection of dyssynergia of the speech apparatus, an *ataxic dysarthria.* An irregular pattern of articulation with a tendency to telescope single or sequential syllables is typical, and a thickened quality is characteristic. *Scanning* speech may be observed in these patients and is characterized by excessive stress on parts of speech that are normally unstressed; slowing of speech and the occurrence of unduly long intervals between phonemes or words, or both, are ordinarily found as well. In parkinsonism a dysarthric defect sometimes referred to as *hypokinetic dysarthria* is encountered. Primarily, the speech is muffled and monotonous in both pitch and loudness; imprecision of articulation, harshness or sibilance, variability in rate, and inappropriate silences may be noted. Patients with chorea and dystonia exhibit excessive variations in loudness and in rate of speech; the term *hyperkinetic dysarthria* is sometimes applied here. In a variety of other conditions, such as general paresis, a simple slurring dysarthria may be found.

Disorders of the *body scheme,* or body image, are particularly common with diseases involving the minor (nondominant) parietal lobe. Unilateral *neglect* (inattention) most frequently affects the left side and may be motor, sensory, or mixed. An example is *dressing apraxia,* in which the patient neglects to dress the left side while clothing himself, but the term is used for any disregard of the left side during voluntary activity. Sensory neglect is brought out by utilizing double simultaneous stimulation (tactile, painful, visual, or auditory); although capable of appreciating these modalities when tested on either side alone, the patient ignores them on the affected side when both sides are tested at the same time. This pattern of neglect may extend to extracorporeal space as well. In a more striking vein, the patient may also be unaware of, or actively deny, the presence of hemiparesis, ordinarily of the left side; this defect is called *anosognosia* (the term is sometimes used in a broader sense to indicate denial of any form of somatic illness). An occasional patient may actually deny the existence of the left side of the body, a state of affairs referred to as *hemisomatotopagnosia* (or amorphosynthesis or hemidepersonalization). In general, disorders of the body scheme are accompanied by alteration of sensation, most importantly proprioception, and by varying degrees of mental confusion. A more subtle defect in the body scheme, not necessarily associated with mental or sensory changes, is right-left disorientation, commonly associated with finger agnosia, dysgraphia, and dyscalculia in the so-called Gerstmann's syndrome; this is observed particularly with lesions involving the dominant parietotemporal region, in contrast to the deficits described hitherto.

CRANIAL NERVES

I. Olfactory

Anosmia, or complete loss of smell, is found most commonly as a result of local disease involving the olfactory bulb, nerve, and tract. It occurs with meningiomas involving the olfactory groove, or with trauma affecting the ethmoid plate, and is associated with laceration of the base of the frontal lobe. It is frequently overlooked by the patient, who may be totally unaware of a complete loss of smell. Hyposmia, or decreased sense of smell, is associated with the same causes as loss of smell but is of little clinical importance since the finding is so common in normal subjects as a result of nasal obstruction, previous catarrh, etc. Repugnant smells are found as a part of uncinate fits in epilepsy and indicate a lesion involving the uncus in the temporal lobe. They are often associated with unpleasant tastes and smacking movements of the lips.

II. Optic

Disease of the optic nerve is characterized by (1) disturbance or loss of visual acuity, (2) visual field defects, (3) changes in the fundus oculi involving the nerve and retina. The optic nerve may be the seat of primary or secondary optic atrophy, the former resulting from direct injury (inflammation, compression, etc.) of the nerve between the retina and optic chiasm, and the latter, from previous infiltration of the nerve that has been replaced by organization of tissue.

Disease of the optic nerve is most frequently associated with partial or complete loss of vision. This is usually slowly progressive in the case of tumors that compress the optic nerves or in such conditions as syphilis or nutritional amblyopia. In other instances, as in acute retrobulbar neuritis, the visual loss is very rapid. In papilledema due to increased intracranial pressure the visual acuity is ordinarily preserved but may deteriorate as secondary ("consecutive") optic atrophy ensues.

VISUAL FIELD DEFECTS. These are found in almost all optic nerve afflictions and in a variety of conditions involving all portions of the visual apparatus. Precise mapping of the visual field abnormality may be of great assistance in localizing cerebral lesions accurately. When the optic nerve is involved anywhere from the retina to the optic chiasm, the visual defect is usually a *scotoma,* which may be central or paracentral or both, the size depending on the degree of nerve damage. With central scotomatous defects there is always loss of visual acuity. Sector defects may be seen, or even unilateral defects obliterating an upper or lower field; such defects, called *altitudinal,* are seen, for example, with subfrontal tumors compressing the optic nerve from above. In disorders involving the optic chiasm, tract, or radiation the defect is *hemianopsia.* These may be *congruous* or *incongruous.* In an incongruous field defect one field is affected more than the other. In a congruous defect they are equally affected.

Hemianopsias may be (1) bitemporal, (2) binasal, or (3) homonymous.

Bitemporal Hemianopsia. This type of hemianopsia is characterized by loss of both temporal fields of vision and is due to compression or disease of the optic chiasm, particularly those fibers decussating within it that are derived from the nasal sides of the retinae. The presence of bitemporal hemianopsia indicates a lesion above the sella turcica. In the majority of instances this lesion is a primary pituitary tumor growing within the sella turcica, expanding upward to compress the optic chiasm. In other instances the condition is due to lesions lying above the sella turcica and compressing the optic chiasm (meningioma, adenoma, craniopharyngioma, aneurysm, arachnoiditis). Parasellar lesions may cause bitemporal hemianopsia by extension medially to compress the chiasm. Bitemporal hemianopsia may in rare instances result from trauma with laceration of the optic chiasm or from pressure by a dilated third ventricle due to internal hydrocephalus from a posterior fossa tumor. The visual field defect in bitemporal hemianopsia is often through the fixation point, involving central vision, but in many instances central vision may be spared. The exact position of the optic chiasm vis-a-vis the sella turcica varies from individual to individual. At times it sits above and somewhat

OS   OD

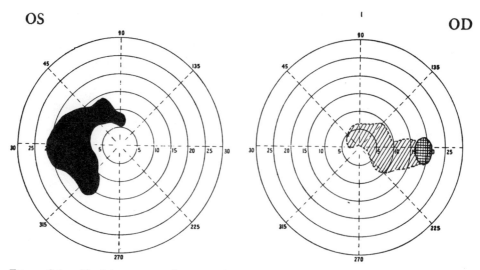

FIGURE 2-1.   Absolute paracentral scotoma in left eye and relative central-paracentral scotoma
in right eye in a patient with multiple sclerosis.

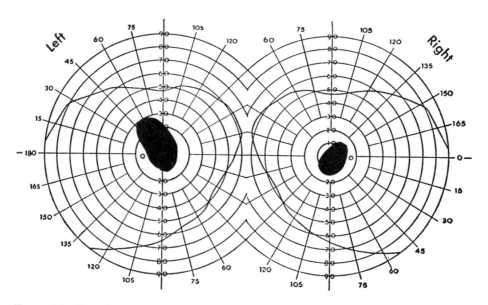

FIGURE 2-2. Central scotomas in a case of multiple sclerosis, with greatly reduced central vision.

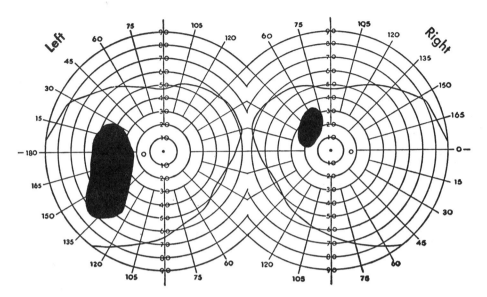

FIGURE 2-3. Paracentral scotomas in both visual fields in a case of multiple sclerosis.

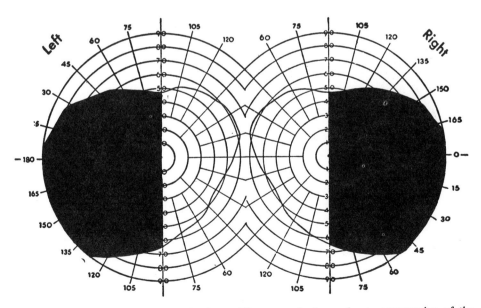

FIGURE 2-4. Bitemporal hemianopsia, in semidiagrammatic form, due to compression of the optic chiasm by a pituitary tumor.

anterior to the sella (pre-fixed chiasm), and at other times above and slightly behind (post-fixed); instead of a pure bitemporal hemianopsia, mixed field abnormalities may appear with suprasellar lesions as a result of such anatomic variation.

Binasal Hemianopsia. A loss of the nasal halves of the field of vision is characteristic of this variety of field cut; it thus comprises the exact opposite of bitemporal hemianopsia. It is produced by lesions that compress the optic chiasm from the sides and is most commonly encountered with fusiform atherosclerotic aneurysms of the internal carotid arteries.

Homonymous Hemianopsia. This is characterized by loss of the temporal field of one eye and of the nasal field of the other. It may involve the entire homonymous half-fields, or less commonly it may produce a quadrantic defect (quadrantanopsia). The field defect may spare or involve central vision. Homonymous hemianopsia results from disease of the optic tract or radiation from the optic chiasm to its termination in the occipital lobe. Involvement of the optic tract, i.e., that portion of the visual system between the chiasm and the lateral geniculate body, is most commonly due to tumors, aneurysms, or trauma. Many conditions can involve the optic radiations beyond the geniculate body in the temporal and occipital lobes, including softening, hemorrhage, tumor, abscess, encephalitis, and multiple sclerosis and other demyelinating diseases. In general, homonymous hemianopsia due to tract lesions is accompanied by pupillary abnormalities, whereas such are not found when the offending lesion is distal to the geniculate body.

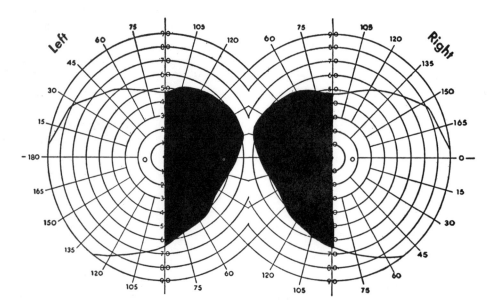

FIGURE 2-5. Binasal hemianopsia, a rare form of visual field defect, in this case due to interruption of the fibers from the temporal sides of the retina by compression from sclerosed internal carotid arteries.

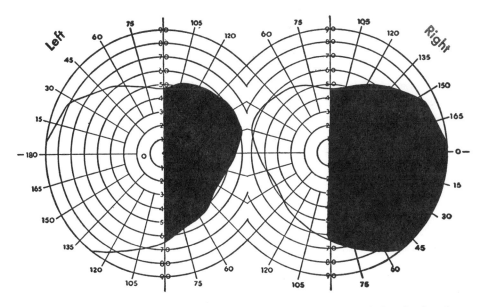

FIGURE 2-6.   Homonymous hemianopsia (right) due to interruption of the visual pathways
in the left temporal lobe in a case of brain tumor.

Differences in the configuration of the visual fields have been used in order
to indicate precise localization, but these have only very limited value. Thus
homonymous field defects through the fixation point are said to indicate temporal
lobe lesions since the fibers are closely packed together here, while defects with
sparing of the fixation point are more likely to be due to occipital lesions. Though
this is true to a limited degree it is not constant. Defects with involvement of
central vision occur often in occipital lobe lesions, and sparing of central vision is
not uncommon with temporal lobe lesions. It is usually asserted that a lesion of
the optic tract can be differentiated from one involving the optic radiation by the
following features: (1) A tract lesion tends to be incongruous, one field being
affected more than the other. This is not constant, but it is true that a tract lesion
is more likely if the fields are incongruous. (2) The macular fibers are affected,
but, as has been pointed out, this may occur in lesions of the radiation if the lesion
is large enough.

Under some circumstances only parts of homonymous visual fields are affected.
Thus, a quadrantic field defect involving either the upper or lower homonymous
quadrants is sometimes seen and is referred to as superior or inferior *quadrantanopsia*. Superior or upper quadrantanopsia is more likely to result from a temporal
lobe lesion due to damage to the lower fibers of the optic radiation. Inferior or
lower quadrantanopsia is more likely to be due to involvement of the upper part
of the radiation in or adjacent to the parietal lobe.

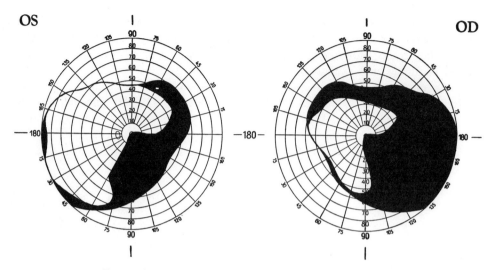

FIGURE 2-7.   Incongruous right homonymous hemianopsia.

Under rare circumstances a lesion of the optic radiation, usually tumor, may produce a crescentic or hemicrescentic defect in the periphery of the temporal field of vision of one eye, without involvement of the homonymous field of the opposite eye. The defect is in the peripheral temporal field, representing the uniocular field of vision. Such field defects usually begin in the periphery and advance toward the center, frequently sparing central vision; they regress in reverse manner.

Concentric contraction of the visual fields is found in patients with greatly decreased vision, and with a variety of disorders involving primarily the neurocellular elements of the retinae. This form of field abnormality is also found in hysteria in the form of tubular vision.

OPTIC NERVE ABNORMALITIES. *Primary Optic Atrophy.* This results from many causes. The important neurological conditions associated with primary optic atrophy are: (1) tumors such as pituitary or suprasellar neoplasms, sphenoid ridge or olfactory groove meningiomas, or aneurysms; (2) inflammations, including tertiary syphilis (tabes dorsalis, general paresis); (3) demyelinating diseases, particularly multiple sclerosis; (4) degenerative conditions such as Friedreich's ataxia or other spinocerebellar degenerations, Leber's hereditary optic atrophy, or primary retinal degenerations such as retinitis pigmentosa; (5) intoxications due to arsenic (tryparsamide), lead, quinine, methyl alcohol, etc.; (6) miscellaneous conditions such as exsanguination, trauma, and anoxia.

Secondary Optic Atrophy. This develops in optic nerves that have been previously inflamed or edematous, in which organization has occurred. It may follow optic or retrobulbar neuritis, choked disc, and vascular obstructions.

Choked Disc or Papilledema. This is characterized by swelling and edema and sometimes hyperemia of the optic nerve head associated with dilatation and tortuosity of the retinal veins. The nerve head is elevated above the level of the retina, the edges of the nerve being first obscured, then completely obliterated. The surrounding retina shows no changes at first, but later hemorrhages appear as the edema continues and exudates may develop as the process becomes older. The elevation of the nerve head in choked disc is measured by first focusing the ophthalmoscope clearly on the retina at some distance from the disc and then focusing on the edematous nerve head itself. The difference between the two readings represents the elevation of the choked disc as measured in diopters of swelling (1D, 2D, etc.). About 3D of swelling is equivalent to 1mm. of elevation of the nerve head.

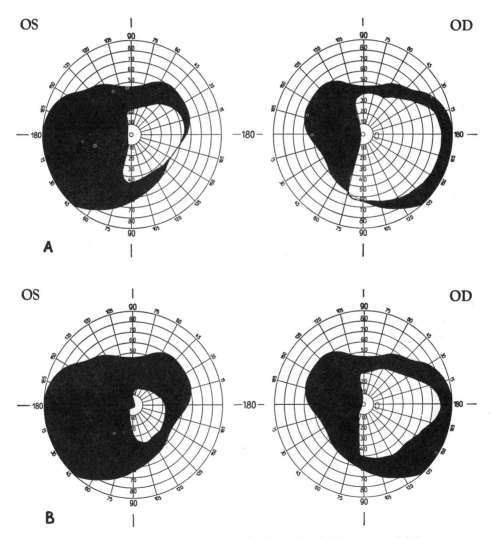

FIGURE 2-8. *A*. Congruous left homonymous hemianopsia. *B*. Incongruous left homonymous hemianopsia.

Because of varying degrees of accommodation on the part of the examiner, the measurement of disc elevation in diopters may be misleading and should not be considered precise. The choked disc eventually becomes organized and replaced by glial tissue, the edema receding and the nerve head becoming visible as gliosis proceeds. Secondary optic atrophy ultimately develops, the nerve head appearing grayish or grayish white, and the edges indistinct in outline.

Choked disc is caused by tumor of the brain in the vast majority of instances, but it may be caused by other conditions that raise intracranial pressure such as subdural hematoma, brain abscess, or chronic meningitis.

The swelling and hyperemia of the disc noted in acute optic neuritis may be confused with true papilledema; ordinarily, a loss of visual acuity and a central scotoma are found with optic neuritis and serve to distinguish this condition from papilledema, in which the visual acuity is normal and the visual fields abnormal only in terms of enlargement of the blind spot. Conditions such as *drusen* or *medullated nerve fibers* may also have to be distinguished from true papilledema, generally with little difficulty.

III, IV, VI. Ocular

Diseases of the ocular nerves produce (1) changes in the pupils, (2) disturbances of ocular movements (ophthalmoplegias).

Abnormalities of the pupils are found in diseases involving the oculomotor nerve. The normal pupil is round, centrally placed, regular in outline, equal in size to its fellow, and responds promptly to light, accommodation, and consensual reactions. Unequal, irregular pupils reacting slowly to light are found in syphilis of the nervous system and occasionally in other conditions. A pupil may be said to be slow and sluggish in its reaction when it contracts slowly or imperfectly to direct light or when after contraction it relaxes almost immediately. The arc of contraction is smaller in sluggishly reacting pupils. *Argyll Robertson pupils* are found in tabes dorsalis particularly and less frequently in other forms of neurosyphilis. They have also been described in encephalitis, multiple sclerosis, infiltrating tumors of the midbrain, chronic alcoholism, and diabetes. Isolated loss of the light reflex (not typical Argyll Robertson pupils) has been described in diabetes mellitus, trauma of the eyeball and orbit, and syringomyelia. Argyll Robertson pupils are characterized by the following features: They are contracted and small in typical cases, irregular in outline, often unequal, and fail to react to light. In typical instances they respond to accommodation, but the reaction may be so slight that it is difficult to see. They respond poorly to painful stimuli and dilate but slightly with mydriatics. Nonreactive dilated pupils are occasionally encountered in luetic persons; strictly speaking they are not typically Argyll Robertson in type. The pupillary abnormality is most commonly bilateral, though unilateral instances are sometimes found. The pathogenesis of the Argyll Robertson pupil is not known. It may be due to interruption of the afferent limb of the reflex arc in the posterior commissure (Merritt and Moore) or to a lesion at the synapses between the cells of the sphincter of the iris and the reflex collaterals surrounding these cells (Spiegel). Unilateral dilated pupil failing to react to light (*Hutchinson's pupil*) is found at times in subdural hematoma and in other instances of increased intracranial pressure with herniation of the uncus of the temporal lobe through the incisura of the tentorium against the third nerve. The phase of dilatation, which is due to parasympathetic paralysis, is ordinarily preceded by a stage of pupillary constriction resulting from parasympathetic irritation early in the course of compression. A similar pupillary dilatation results from irritation of the cervical sympathetic pathway from its peripheral course in the neck to its central portion.

Horner's syndrome is the result of paralysis of the cervical sympathetic outflow and is characterized by contraction of the pupil, partial ptosis of the eyelid, enophthalmos and, inconstantly, loss of sweating over the affected side of the face. It may be due to (1) lesions affecting the cervical sympathetic trunk in the neck, e.g., gunshot or stab wounds, disease of the cervical glands, tumors, aneurysms; (2) spinal cord (segments C8 to T1) or root (C8 to T1) lesions: extramedullary such as tumors, trauma, pachymeningitis, and intramedullary such as syringomyelia, tumors, hematomyelia, syphilitic meningomyelitis; (3) brain stem lesions, particularly in the medulla, such as syringomyelia, softenings, and infiltrating tumors.

Paradoxical pupil is characterized by dilation of the pupil on stimulation by light. It is found at times in tabes dorsalis.

The *tonic pupil* of *Adie's syndrome* is usually found in women, is often unilateral (80 per cent), and is usually larger than its fellow. It responds poorly and slowly to light; in the dark the pupil dilates, after which it responds to light and reacts normally to mydriatics. It may be associated with loss of the Achilles or patellar reflex, or both. The most important feature of the myotonic pupil is its behavior on convergence. "If the patient fixes a near object and continues to gaze at it intently, the pupil, sometimes after a delay of several seconds, contracts slowly and with increasing slowness through a range, often greatly in excess of the normal; contraction down to pinhead size is not uncommon; the large abnormal pupil then becomes smaller than its fellow" (Adie). It has been found that the abnormal pupil manifests marked constriction after instillation of 2.5 per cent methacholine, while the normal pupil fails to react.

Disturbances of movement of the eyeballs are found regularly in disease involving the ocular nerves. These are spoken of as *opthalmoplegias*. The nerves (III, IV, VI) may be involved either singly or in unison in neurological diseases. They may be affected (1) within the brain stem by involvement of their nuclei; (2) peripherally in their course at the base of the brain; (3) within the orbit. Within the brain stem they may be affected by infiltrating tumors, multiple sclerosis, encephalitis of various sorts, hemorrhage, softening, or in such metabolic diseases as Wernicke's encephalopathy. At the base of the brain they may be involved in meningitis of various types, particularly syphilitic; subarachnoid hemorrhage; aneurysms of the internal carotid, posterior communicating or posterior cerebral arteries; meningiomas of the sphenoid ridge; trauma; neuritis due to such causes as lead or diabetes; extension of nasopharyngeal carcinoma; and mastoid disease resulting in petrositis and affecting especially the abducens nerve (*Gradenigo syndrome*).

COMPLETE PARALYSIS OF ALL OCULAR NERVES. This results in ptosis of the eyelids and complete immobility of the eyeballs, which cannot be moved in any direction (*external ophthalmoplegia*). The pupils are dilated and do not react to light because of paralysis of the sphincter iridis and over-reaction of the cervical sympathetics (*internal ophthalmoplegia*). Such paralysis may be unilateral or bilateral, more frequently the former. It is more likely to be the result of involvement of the nerves themselves than of their nuclei in the brain stem. Complete paralysis of all the ocular nerves is produced usually by lesions in the region of the cavernous sinus, where all the nerves are concentrated in a small area on their way to their respective muscles in the eyeball. The syndrome may be produced by meningitis, thrombosis of the cavernous sinus, or by tumors or aneurysms compressing the cavernous sinus; it may also be produced by lesions within the orbit itself. It is less often associated with lesions within the brain stem. Disorders such as myasthenia gravis or ocular myopathy may result in complete external ophthalmoplegia, but the pupils are spared.

Partial paralysis of the ocular nerves may occur in various combinations either unilaterally or bilaterally and may be due to a variety of causes similar to those involving all the nerves. Partial paralyses are more likely to be due to lesions within the brain stem, particularly if other signs of involvement of cranial nerve or other intramedullary systems are present. Diplopia is characteristic of partial paralyses, the pattern of double vision being dependent on the particular nerves and muscles involved.

ISOLATED PARALYSIS OF THE OCULOMOTOR (III) NERVE. Bilateral complete paralysis of the oculomotor nerve is rare but may follow arteriosclerotic softening involving the nuclei in the midbrain, encephalitis, or multiple sclerosis. The eyes are held in a divergent squint, the pupils are dilated, there is bilateral ptosis, and the eyeballs cannot be moved upward, inward, or downward.

Unilateral complete paralysis is more common and is usually due to compression of the nerve by aneurysm of the internal carotid or posterior communicating artery, by tumor of the sphenoid ridge, by extension of a pituitary tumor, by meningitis, meningeal hemorrhage involving the nerve in the interpeduncular space, trauma, or penetrating wounds of the orbit. It commonly appears as a cranial mononeuropathy with diabetes. It is less likely to be the result of brain stem affection.

The condition is characterized by dilatation of the pupil, ptosis of the eyelid with inability to open the lid, external strabismus resulting from the unopposed pull of the external rectus muscle, and inability to move the affected eyeball upward, inward, or downward. Reaction of the pupil to light is lost. In most instances the pupil is dilated and fixed, but it may not be dilated, and there are some cases of compressive syndrome due to aneurysm with pupillary escape, i.e., retention of the pupillary reaction. Involvement in diabetic ophthalmoplegia characteristically spares the pupil as well.

Incomplete paralyses involving the oculomotor nerve may be due to either intramedullary or extramedullary factors. Loss or impairment of convergence is found without other evidence of oculomotor paralysis as a residual of epidemic encephalitis. Isolated muscles innervated by the oculomotor nerve may be involved selectively in brain stem disease, since the various muscles innervated by the oculomotor nerves have specific localizations within the oculomotor nucleus. Iso-

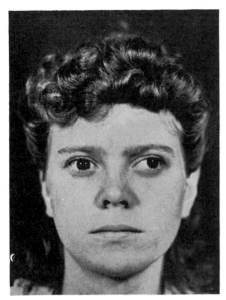
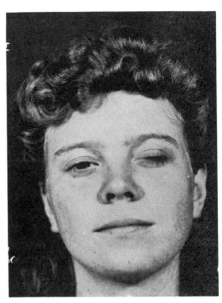

FIGURE 2-9. Partial ophthalmoplegia, with involvement of the left oculomotor nerve, showing the ptosis of the eyelid and external strabismus in a case of cerebral aneurysm.

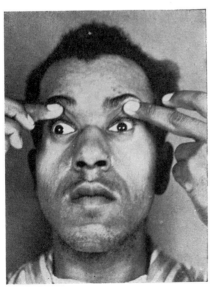
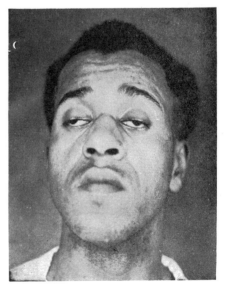

FIGURE 2-10. Partial ophthalmoplegia involving the oculomotor nerve bilaterally and showing ptosis, paralysis of upward movement of the eyeballs, and bilateral external strabismus due to the unopposed action of both external rectus muscles.

lated muscle paralyses may occur also from compression of the nerve itself by aneurysm, tumor, syphilitic meningitis, etc.

ISOLATED PARALYSIS OF THE TROCHLEAR (IV) NERVE. This is not a common condition in neurological practice but is frequently seen in ophthalmological practice. The responsible lesions may be in the brain stem or in the nerve itself. The trochlear nerve innervates the superior oblique muscle and moves the eyeball downward and outward; with the globe directed mesially, it is responsible for downward movement with intorsion. This movement is lost in paralysis of the nerve. Tilting of the head toward the shoulder is a constant accompanying sign. This posture permits binocular vision without diplopia, the latter developing as soon as the head is held in the vertical position. Because of the head tilt, cases of trochlear paralysis are frequently mistaken for torticollis and are often treated as such for a long time before the correct diagnosis is made.

ISOLATED PARALYSIS OF THE ABDUCENS (VI) NERVE. The abducens nerve innervates the external rectus muscle. Paralysis of the nerve results in inability to rotate the eyeball outward. This is readily recognized by the internal squint due to the unopposed action of the internal rectus muscle. Diplopia is present, and the head is turned in the direction in which the eye muscle had been acting before it was paralyzed. Abducens paralysis is due to a variety of causes, most of which have already been discussed. It may be involved in lesions of the cavernous sinus, trauma, meningitis, meningeal hemorrhage, and in infection of the petrous bone in mastoid disease associated with pain in the face and eye (Gradenigo syndrome). Of particular interest is its occurrence as a nonspecific sign of increased intracranial pressure. A study of the causes of 104 cases of abducens paralysis is shown in Figure 2-11. It is apparent that the cause cannot always be determined.

CONJUGATE PARALYSES. Paralyses of conjugate movement of the eyes occur under diverse circumstances. Their identification is often extremely useful in localizing lesions to the brain stem or cerebral hemispheres. To permit full evaluation, examination should include the following: (1) volitional movements; (2) attraction movements, consisting of quick movements of the eyes toward an object in the periphery that attracts the attention; (3) following movements; (4) segmental reflex movements (oculocephalic, caloric).

Paralysis of lateral gaze consists of inability to move the eyeballs voluntarily laterally in a horizontal plane. Despite this loss of voluntary movement, the eyeballs can sometimes follow a directing finger to the paralyzed side. Paralysis of lateral gaze may result from a lesion in the pons, where a center is presumed to exist for such conjugate movement, in the para-abducens area, or from involvement of the supranuclear centers for conjugate gaze in the cerebrum (located in the so-called adversive eye field of the opposite frontal lobe and in the occipital lobe). Conjugate deviation of the eyes in cerebral lesions may be encountered in both irritative and destructive lesions. In *irritative* lesions, the eyes deviate to the opposite side, i.e., they look away from the lesion, whereas in *destructive* lesions they gaze toward the side of the lesion because of the unopposed action of the centers in the opposite hemisphere.

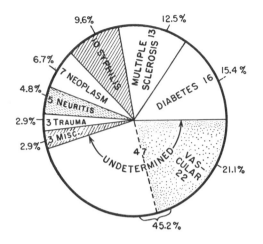

FIGURE 2-11. Abducens nerve paralysis. Diagnostic classification. (From Shrader, E. C., and Schlezinger, N. S.: Neuro-ophthalmologic Evaluation of Abducens Paralysis. Arch. Ophthal. 63:84, 1960.)

The distinction between supranuclear and pontine paralysis of lateral gaze is often difficult. The following points are helpful: (a) The presence of accessory signs may indicate whether a cerebral or brain stem lesion is responsible for the paralysis of lateral gaze. Thus, absence of the corneal reflex and the occurrence of motor paralysis of the trigeminal nerve, abducens paralysis, or facial paralysis point to a pontine lesion; (b) in pontine lesions, the eyes are unable to follow the directing finger; in cerebral lesions this can often be done; (c) the paralysis in a pontine lesion is permanent, while that of a cerebral lesion is transitory; (d) segmental reflex movements are commonly lost with pontine lesions and preserved with cerebral lesions. Under the latter circumstance, qualitative changes such as directional preponderance may appear.

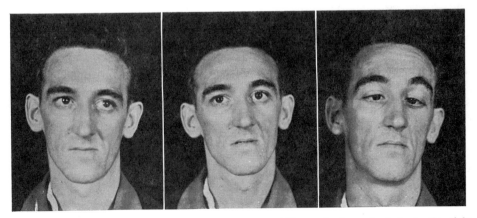

FIGURE 2-12. Paralysis of lateral gaze. Note the inability to look particularly to the right and the loss of near convergence with the right eye.

Paralysis of upward gaze (*Parinaud syndrome*) is characterized by inability to move the eyeballs upward above the horizontal plane. It is usually though not always associated with paralysis of downward gaze as well. It frequently exists without evidence of involvement of other ocular muscles but is often associated with changes in the pupillary reactions. It is rarely found as an isolated symptom. The syndrome is found in tumors of the pineal body, in infiltrating tumors of the collicular plate (superior colliculus), in Wernicke's encephalopathy, softenings, and, rarely, as a distant symptom due to pressure from cerebellopontine angle or cerebellar tumor. Its exact cause is not known. It is thought to be due to pressure or invasion of the superior colliculi, perhaps with involvement of the central gray matter around the aqueduct of Sylvius. Irritation in the same area is presumably responsible for the forced upward gaze of the *oculogyric crises* of postencephalitic parkinsonism.

Paralysis of divergence is extremely difficult to determine. A center for divergence has not been conclusively demonstrated. Divergence paralysis is characterized by the following: (a) homonymous diplopia; (b) failure of increase of the angle of squint on looking to the right or left, but increase (or decrease) on looking downward and upward; as a result, the head in some cases is held with the chin against the chest in order to promote convergence; (c) approach of the images closer to one another on bringing a test object close to the patient, and fusion at 10 to 15 inches from the patient; (d) the development of further diplopia when the test object is brought within this area because of the failure of convergence; (e) preservation of function of the lateral recti. There is much doubt on the part of some as to whether divergence paralysis is a true condition.

Paralysis of convergence is characterized by loss of ability of the eyeballs to converge on near objects, with normal function of the individual medial recti. It is found in encephalitis lethargica, which has a predilection for involving the oculomotor nerve complex and particularly the nucleus of convergence, and in parkinsonism of both the postencephalitic and idiopathic varieties. It is also encountered in old age and with softenings and multiple sclerosis. Paralysis of movement of the internal rectus muscles with *retention* of convergence is designated as *internuclear ophthalmoplegia* and is due to a lesion involving the medial longitudinal fasciculus (posterior longitudinal bundle). It is found most commonly in multiple sclerosis; unilateral instances are often due to softenings. Characteristically associated with the paralysis of adduction is nystagmus of the abducting eye, so-called ataxic nystagmus. *Convergence spasms* may occur under a variety of circumstances, such as multiple sclerosis, but are most frequently hysterical in origin.

V. Trigeminal

The trigeminal nerve is composed of both motor and sensory portions; hence motor and sensory manifestations may be found alone or in combination. Atrophy of the affected masseter and temporal can be detected by palpation of the muscles directly; weakness can be elicited as already described (Chapter 1). It will be recalled that deviation of the jaw is toward the paralyzed side when the mouth is

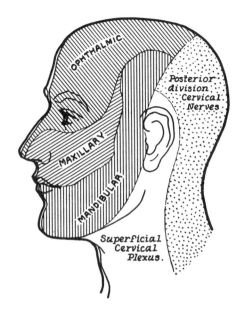

FIGURE 2-13. Trigeminal nerve, showing the areas of supply of the three
principal divisions.

opened. Because of the deflection of the jaw the tongue appears to be deviated as
well, but this is not the case, since a line drawn through the incisors will be found
to cut through the tip of the tongue.

Weakness involving the masseter, temporal, and pterygoids, which are supplied
by the trigeminal nerve, may be the result of a peripheral lesion such as trauma,
skull fracture, or tumor. It may also result from a tumor of the cerebellopontine
angle that compresses the trigeminal nerve at its exit from the pons or from an

FIGURE 2-14. Trigeminal nerve, showing the type of onion-peel sensory
loss (pain and temperature) found in
lesions within the brain stem affecting
the descending root of the trigeminal
nerve.

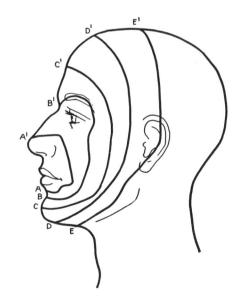

infiltrating tumor or other lesion of the pons involving the motor nucleus of the trigeminal nerve.

The sensory division of the trigeminal nerve supplies the face and head to the vertex, the cornea, and the mucous membranes of the nose, mouth, hard and soft palate, and tongue to the midline. Complete interruption of sensory function is rare but occurs with tumors of the gasserian ganglion or with inflammatory disease of this ganglion such as herpes. In such instances it is associated with pain in the face along the branches of the trigeminal nerve. Incomplete sensory syndromes involving the face are found in infiltrating tumors of the pons, or with other conditions that affect the sensory trigeminal nucleus, such as multiple sclerosis or softening. In general, the sensory loss under these circumstances is in the distribution of one or another of the classical peripheral divisions of the nerve. It must be remembered that there is reversal of representation in the descending (spinal) root of the trigeminal, the ophthalmic division (V_1) being represented most inferiorly, the mandibular (V_3) and maxillary (V_2) divisions more superiorly. Lesions higher in the tract in the brain stem may thus give rise to a sensory deficit over the lower face, while a lesion low in the medulla may be associated with sensory loss over the forehead. On occasion, however, a special variety of sensory alteration is encountered with lesions of the descending root: The sensory loss may follow a so-called onion-peel arrangement, not corresponding to the accustomed anatomical zones in the periphery. Direct involvement of the peripheral branches of the trigeminal nerve may be due to many circumstances, including tumor, infection such as herpes, and trauma. Involvement of the ophthalmic division with disease of the cavernous sinus is noteworthy.

One of the early manifestations of sensory loss of the trigeminal nerve is impairment of the corneal reflex. This may be the only manifestation of involvement of the sensory branch. It occurs early in many cases of cerebellopontine angle tumor. It is found in hemiplegia, in thalamic syndromes, in infiltrating tumor of the pons, encephalitis, multiple sclerosis, tumor of the gasserian ganglion, herpes zoster ophthalmicus, after section of the trigeminal nerve for trigeminal neuralgia, and in any disorder affecting the gasserian ganglion, the sensory nucleus of the trigeminal nerve in the pons, or in local conditions of the eye.

Although the trigeminal nerve plays an important role in autonomic function, abnormalities in this sphere are only rarely encountered with trigeminal nerve dysfunction. A Horner's syndrome in association with facial pain may, however, be seen as the so-called *paratrigeminal syndrome,* which is usually due to extra-medullary tumor or aneurysm.

VII. Facial

Involvement of the facial nerve occurs frequently in disease of the nervous system. Careful distinction must be made between central and peripheral nerve involvement.

Central facial weakness is characterized by weakness of movement of the lower portion of the face on the side opposite the lesion, movements of the frontalis being preserved. This sparing is due to the fact that the upper portions of the face receive innervation from both motor areas; the lower portion is innervated only from the opposite motor cortex. It is recognized by a slight drooping of the corner of the mouth and upper lip on the affected side during repose, flattening of the nasolabial fold, and weakness in retraction of the corner of the mouth on the affected side. Slight differences require careful scrutiny and are sometimes difficult to recognize. In the usual case of central facial weakness the forehead can be wrinkled normally and closure of the eyelid is normal. In acute cases, however, a slight weakness in wrinkling the forehead and in closing the eye may be seen; in such instances the weakness in the lower portion of the face is always more pro-

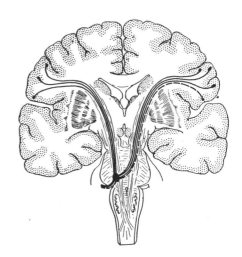

FIGURE 2-15. Facial nerve illustrating the bilateral innervation of the upper portion of the facial nerve (solid lines) and the unilateral innervation of the lower portion (broken lines), thus accounting for sparing of the frontalis muscle in central facial weakness.

nounced, while that of the upper portions tends to disappear within a few days as a rule. While voluntary facial expression due to a hemispheral lesion is weak in central palsies, emotional expression remains intact or may even be exaggerated. In lesions of the thalamus, however, emotional expression may be lost, while voluntary movements are intact. This dissociation of voluntary and emotional expression may be important in differentiating a deep-seated from a cortical lesion.

Weakness of central type may result from lesions involving the motor innervation to the face anywhere between the face area in the opposite motor cortex and the nucleus of the facial nerve in the pons. It may be isolated or associated with weakness of the hand, arm, or other parts of the body. Central facial weakness existing alone, or with other focal weakness (faciobrachial monoplegia, etc.), is usually the result of a small focal lesion of the opposite motor cortex but may be a residual of an old hemiplegia. In most instances central facial weakness is associated with hemiplegia and is due to simultaneous interruption of corticospinal and corticobulbar pathways by a wide variety of pathological processes.

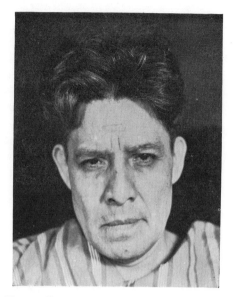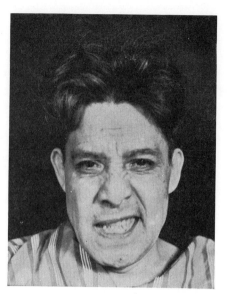

FIGURE 2-16. Central facial weakness showing the drooping of the right corner of the mouth
with the face in repose and the weakness of retraction of the mouth on voluntary effort.

Peripheral facial paralysis differs from central facial weakness by virtue of
the involvement of all portions of the facial musculature. It results from a lesion
of the facial nerve anywhere along its peripheral course from the facial nucleus
in the pons to its distribution in the face. The lesion producing the paralysis is
ipsilateral to the paralysis. All portions of the face on the affected side are paralyzed.
Wrinkling of the forehead, closure of the eyelid, and movements of the muscles of

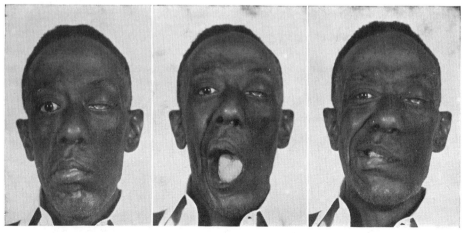

FIGURE 2-17. Peripheral facial paralysis showing the involvement of all facial muscles of the
left side, with inability to wrinkle the forehead and to close the eyelid and paralysis of the
muscles of facial expression.

facial expression are impossible; taste is at times lost on the anterior two thirds of the tongue on the affected side; the nerve trunks of the face may be tender. Peripheral facial paralysis may result from involvement of the facial nucleus or the intramedullary portion of the nerve in the pons as in poliomyelitis, encephalitis, softening, or infiltrating tumors of the pons. It may be involved as a result of disease of the nerve within the skull, as in cerebellopontine angle tumors, meningitis (syphilitic, tuberculous), sarcoidosis, or subarachnoid hemorrhage, or it may ensue from disease of the facial nerve at any point after its emergence from the skull as the result of neuritis, fracture of the skull, tumors of the neck, herpes zoster, etc. Paralysis resulting from involvement of the facial nucleus is characterized by signs of anterior horn cell involvement—atrophy of the muscle and fasciculations—in addition to paralysis. Involvement of the nerve trunk is featured by the usual signs of affection of a motor nerve; a loss of taste over the anterior two thirds of the tongue is found when the nerve is diseased in the mastoid canal.

VIII. Acoustic

The acoustic nerve is composed of *cochlear* and *vestibular* divisions, the former having to do with hearing, the latter with equilibrium. Disease of the cochlea is characterized by nerve or perceptive deafness, the main features of which are loss or impairment of hearing, loss of air conduction, and failure to lateralize sound to the affected ear. Usually there is an associated history of tinnitus, but this is sometimes lacking. Tinnitus may be present for some time before deafness ensues.

Tinnitus is usually the result of disease of the end-organ and is associated with middle or inner ear disease or with disease of the peripheral portions of the auditory nerve. Rarely it develops as a consequence of involvement of the central projections of the auditory nerve in the brain stem. The constancy and nature of the tinnitus are of no help clinically in distinguishing a peripheral from a central origin.

Nerve deafness is practically always the result of disease of the peripheral portion of the auditory nerve. Theoretically, it may occur as a result of central lesions involving the auditory pathways in the brain stem and their termination in the temporal lobe. Actually this occurs extremely rarely because of the fact that the auditory pathways are both crossed and uncrossed; a very extensive lesion would be required to cause loss of hearing. Loss of hearing may be tested much more accurately by the audiometer than by tuning-fork tests. By this means, notes of standard pitch and varying intensities are sent through the ear. Nerve deafness is indicated by a loss of hearing in the higher frequencies. A special form of hearing disturbance is found in *Meniere's disease,* consisting of distortion of sound in the affected ear, hyperacusis, diplacusis, and loudness recruitment.

The vestibular portion of the auditory nerve is frequently affected in diseases of the nervous system. Its outstanding feature is vertigo, a subjective sensation requiring careful analysis.

NYSTAGMUS. This is found in disease of the vestibular portion of the auditory nerve, as well as in other conditions. A consideration of its features is desirable at this point.

Definition. Nystagmus is an involuntary oscillation of the eyeball. It is usually bilateral, the two eyes moving synchronously, but unilateral dysconjugate nystagmus may occur. It may be rhythmical or pendular. In rhythmical nystagmus, there are alternate slow and quick ocular movements, the rapid movement being in the direction of gaze, followed by a slower return movement. In pendular nystagmus, there are more or less regular to-and-fro movements of equal range and velocity.

Nystagmus may be horizontal, vertical, oblique, rotatory, or mixed in form and may be directed to the right, left, upward, or downward. It may be slow, medium, or fast and may vary from 10 to 1000 oscillations per minute. It may be transient or sustained, congenital or acquired, spontaneous or induced, and may be present at rest, on fixation, or on deviation of the eyeballs.

The slow, or following, phase of nystagmus seems the primary event and is dependent on the visual act. Integrity of the occipital cortex is essential for its appearance, and the movement is probably mediated by the so-called optomotor field of the occipital lobes. The fast phase is correctional or compensatory, is closely akin to rotary eye movements, and may be controlled by frontal or vestibular mechanisms, possibly both. Traditionally, nystagmus is named after the direction of the fast component, even though that is probably of secondary rather than primary significance.

Classification of Nystagmus. Many classifications have been utilized in attempting to clarify the problem of nystagmus. A common grouping, for example, is into

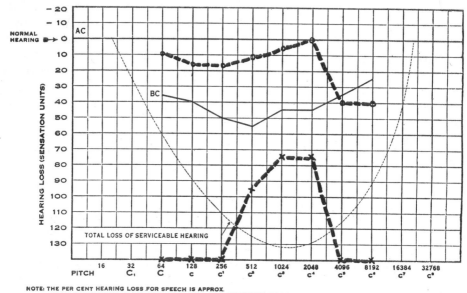

FIGURE 2-18. Audiometer chart. There is a characteristic nerve deafness involving the left ear as revealed by the loss of hearing of the higher frequencies.

ocular, vestibular, and central types. It may be graded on the basis of severity, with first degree (nystagmus present only on gaze to one side), second degree (present on gaze to one side and directly ahead), and third degree (present on gaze to both sides, as well as straight ahead). The approach utilized here follows Cogan in most particulars; it has the advantage of being based directly on the characteristics of the movements as they are seen by the examiner.

1. Pendular nystagmus

The movements are oscillating, almost always horizontal, and approximately equal in both directions; only one eye may be involved, and under these circumstances the movements may be vertical. Head nodding may accompany the eye movements. When the patient looks to either side, jerk (or rhythmical) nystagmus appears with the fast component in the direction of gaze. Impairment of central vision is a hallmark of pendular variety of nystagmus, and the worse the vision the coarser are the movements. Pendular nystagmus is characteristically encountered in individuals with vision defective from birth or infancy or in those with defective fixation. If vision is lost after the age of 6 years, no such movements occur. The term "searching" is sometimes applied to this form of nystagmus, with the connotation that the eyes are moving to compensate for the central scotoma that is generally present; this does not seem to be the case, however, and the movements more likely result from failure of normal tonic innervation of the ocular muscles from the macula. Many conditions are associated with pendular nystagmus, including infantile macular choreoretinitis, albinism with faulty development of the macula, total color blindness, congenital cataract, ophthalmia neonatorum, interstitial keratitis, congenital corneal leukoma, and high-grade infantile myopia.

Several subvarieties of pendular nystagmus may be isolated:

a. Occupational nystagmus. This is oscillating, fine, rapid, often vertical, and increased on upward gaze. Fixation is defective. It is seen in miners and in others who work in poor light for long periods, such as compositors, draftsmen, jewelers, train dispatchers, crane workers, and painters.

b. Spasmus nutans. Usually associated with head nodding, and either monocular or binocular, this form of pendular nystagmus is rapid and often asymmetrical, varying with different directions of gaze. It generally appears within the first 2 years of life and ordinarily disappears spontaneously. Although sometimes likened to occupational nystagmus, its cause is unknown.

c. Voluntary nystagmus. Some individuals are able to induce very rapid horizontal oscillating movements of the eyes on a voluntary basis. Fixation, convergence, or widening of the palpebral fissures may increase the movements. Similar movements, associated with rigid fixation of the head, may be seen in neurotic individuals.

2. Jerk nystagmus (rhythmical nystagmus)

In this form of nystagmus the movements are unequal, and both fast and slow components can be recognized. As already indicated, the nystagmus is named after the fast component, even though this is probably secondary from the pathogenetic standpoint.

a. Optokinetic nystagmus. Generally rather fine and rapid, horizontal in plane, this form of nystagmus is elicited by rotating a drum with vertical stripes before the eyes; it also occurs when a person on a rapidly moving vehicle directs his eyes on fixed objects (railroad or elevator nystagmus). The slow, or following, phase is in the direction of rotation of the drum. Defective opticokinetic responses or absence of them is most commonly found with lesions in the posterior half of the cerebral hemisphere when the drum is rotated to the side of the lesion; thus, the slow phase is impaired. This abnormality may be seen with or without an associated hemianopic defect. More anteriorly placed lesions only uncommonly are associated with this form of abnormality. Bilateral reduction in opticokinetic responses is sometimes found but cannot be correlated accurately with lesions in a particular location.

b. Labyrinthine (vestibular) nystagmus. Characteristically, this follows stimulation of the semicircular canals and results from movement of the endolymph with stimulation of the vestibular nerves. It is characterized by the presence of slow and fast components and may be looked upon as a reflex response to movements of the head or body or to direct stimulation of the labyrinth. It may be horizontal, rotary, or both. Rotation in a Barany chair, thermal (caloric) stimulation, and galvanic excitation may all be utilized to produce this form of nystagmus. Labyrinthine nystagmus may also occur spontaneously in disease of the labyrinth itself or of the vestibular nuclei; spontaneous rotary nystagmus is especially common with lesions affecting the latter structures. When the nystagmus is due to a lesion in the labyrinth (as in labyrinthitis or Meniere's disease) or in the eighth nerve, vertigo, tinnitus, and alteration of hearing are frequent, whereas with central lesions these are uncommon. Loss of response to thermal stimuli is found with nuclear lesions, a feature of major importance in locating the site of involvement. Many pathological processes involve the vestibular nuclei and are thus capable of producing labyrinthine nystagmus; among the more common are softenings with occlusive vascular disease, multiple sclerosis, Wernicke's encephalopathy, and tumors in the cerebellum or cerebellopontine angle. Lesions that involve the medial longitudinal fasciculus (most commonly multiple sclerosis) produce predominantly monocular (ataxic) nystagmus as part of the syndrome of internuclear ophthalmoplegia; this consists of weakness of the medial rectus on conjugate lateral gaze with nystagmus of labyrinthine type in the abducting eye. This is ordinarily bilateral, but unilateral cases are encountered. The nystagmus that may appear in association with lesions of the upper cervical cord may also reflect involvement of the medial longitudinal fasciculus in its lowermost extent.

A variety of chemical substances may produce spontaneous labyrinthine nystagmus or alter induced labyrinthine responses; among these are barbiturates, diphenylhydantoin, quinine, and streptomycin.

In severe instances of labyrinthine nystagmus the patient may experience a sensation of illusory movement of the environment; this is called *oscillopsia*.

c. Nystagmus due to neuromuscular insufficiency. Unsustained nystagmoid jerks are seen in a large number of normal persons on extreme deviation of the eyes. This is referred to as end-position nystagmus and has no clinical significance. Exaggerations of this type of nystagmus are seen in the following:

(1) Paretic nystagmus, which develops on attempts to use a paretic ocular muscle; it may occur with gaze palsies as well.

(2) Fatigue nystagmus, which follows excessive use or increased fatigability of certain ocular muscles.

(3) Nystagmus of eccentric fixation. This occurs on deviation of the eyes beyond the limits of the binocular field. It is jerky and occurs in 50 to 60 per cent of normal individuals.

d. Congenital nystagmus. This dates from birth and is sometimes inherited. It must be differentiated from pendular nystagmus, which does not develop until fixation is attempted. Defective opticokinetic responses may be found.

e. Latent nystagmus. This appears on covering one eye in subjects with poor visual acuity or without binocular vision, especially patients with amblyopia resulting from strabismus. It occurs in the covered eye and is in the direction of the open eye. Its cause is unknown.

f. Positional nystagmus. Often associated with vertigo, this variety of nystagmus has a special significance. It is induced as follows: The patient sits on a table with the head turned to one side and the gaze fixed on the examiner's head. The examiner grasps the patient's head and pushes him back briskly into the supine position with the head below the level of the table and rotated 30 to 45 degrees to one side. If nystagmus occurs the head is held in this position for 30 seconds, after which the patient is brought upright, and the test is repeated with the head turned to the opposite side. In the fatigable type the nystagmus appears after a latency of 2 to 10 seconds and subsides in 5 to 30 seconds. In the nonfatigable type the nystagmus appears without latency, as soon as the head is put in the critical position, and persists as long as this position is maintained. The fatigable type is most common with lesions of the end-organ and is often found after head injuries; the nonfatigable type tends to occur with central lesions.

g. See-saw nystagmus. A rare form of nystagmus, this is characterized by rotary (torsional) movements of the eyes along with dissociated and simultaneous vertical movements; as one eye moves up, the other moves down, and vice versa. It most commonly occurs in cases of suprasellar tumors involving the third ventricle but may also be a result of softening in the upper brain stem.

Several varieties of abnormal eye movements are sometimes confused with nystagmus. *Opsoclonus* consists of irregular and nonrhythmical jerking movements of the eyes encountered in comatose patients with lesions of the brain stem. *Ocular myoclonus* is a syndrome of regular, rhythmical, usually conjugate movements of the eyes, with a frequency between 120 and 140 beats a minute, associated with synchronous movements of the palate and, on occasion, other bulbar muscles. It generally follows a lesion, most commonly softening, interrupting the dentato-rubro-olivary circuit, particularly in the pons. *Ocular dysmetria,* or ocular past-pointing, is literally overshooting of the eyes when directed quickly to a target; it is found with cerebellar disease and is analogous to hypermetria of the limbs. *Oculogyric crises* are found almost always in instances of postencephalitic parkinsonism and consist of attacks of involuntary forced upward deviation of the eyes, at times temporarily controllable with maximal voluntary effort. Abrupt spontaneous conjugate vertical eye movements, generally associated with a loss of lateral movements of the eyes, are referred to as *ocular bobbing*. Most commonly found in comatose individuals, this phenomenon is generally attributed to vascular lesions within the pontine tegmentum with resultant dissociation of vertical from lateral movements. *Nystagmus retractorius* comprises jerk-like retraction movements of the globes, commonly rhythmical, usually bilateral, and occurring either spontaneously or in response to eye movements. Ocular palsies, especially of upward gaze (Parinaud's syndrome), may be found. The responsible lesion appears to reside in the periaqueductal region of the midbrain.

IX. Glossopharyngeal

A lesion involving the glossopharyngeal nerve is characterized by loss of taste over the posterior third of the tongue and impaired sensation over the palate and pharynx. This has been observed in syphilitic meningitis, in infiltrating tumors of the brain stem, and with basal skull fractures. Pain in the throat is found in *glossopharyngeal neuralgia,* a rare disease characterized by severe paroxysms of pain initiated by swallowing. As regards motor function, the glossopharyngeal innervates the stylopharyngeus muscle, which elevates and widens the pharynx in swallowing; impairment is ordinarily not recognizable clinically.

X. Vagus

The vagus is a very long nerve that may be affected in the medulla, at the base of the brain, the jugular foramen, in the neck or thorax, or even in the abdomen. Generally speaking, the vagus on the motor side supplies the musculature of the larynx, pharynx, and palate (external laryngeal, recurrent laryngeal, pharyngeal nerves). It supplies also visceromotor fibers to the heart, lungs, and alimentary tract. It carries sensory impressions from pharynx, larynx, epiglottis, trachea, esophagus, heart, lungs, stomach, and small intestine. Symptoms vary, depending upon the point at which it is involved. From a practical viewpoint, disturbances of swallowing and phonation are the most important.

Within the brain stem, the nerve may be involved by a variety of processes, such as infiltrating tumors, multiple sclerosis, syringomyelia, encephalitis, poliomyelitis, softenings, as with thrombosis of the posterior inferior cerebellar artery, progressive bulbar palsy, amyotrophic lateral sclerosis, and other disorders. Within the cranium it may be involved by tumors, by aneurysms of the vertebral or basilar arteries, fractures of the base of the skull, and syphilitic or other chronic meningitis. In the neck it is subject to injury by stab or gunshot wounds, operations on the thyroid or other neck structures, tumors and aneurysms of the carotid or subclavian arteries. Enlarged glands, tumors, and aortic aneurysms may involve the nerve in the mediastinum.

Aphonia or *hoarseness* may result from involvement of the nucleus ambiguus, of the vagus itself in the medulla or in the posterior fossa, or from recurrent laryngeal paralysis. It is associated with abductor paralysis of the vocal cord, which may be unilateral or bilateral. When the former, hoarseness is noted; when the latter, the voice is lost entirely, and dyspnea and stridorous respirations ensue.

Weakness or paralysis of swallowing (*dysphagia*) occurs under a variety of circumstances. It may be found in hemiplegia and is associated in these circumstances with paralysis or weakness of the soft palate. It may result also from involvement of the muscles of deglutition due to a lesion of the nucleus ambiguus. In such instances the palate moves poorly, and there is loss of power of the middle and inferior constrictors of the pharynx. Regurgitation of food through the nose occurs as a result of inability to close the pharynx on swallowing. In some instances of difficulty in swallowing the palate is capable of moving well while the inferior pharyngeal constrictors fail to function. Loss of function of the latter is seen in weakness or loss of movement of the Adam's apple in attempted swallowing.

Along with these difficulties in speaking and swallowing, lesions of the vagus are also expressed by loss of the palatal and pharyngeal reflexes and by impairment of sensation in the external auditory meatus and the pinna.

XI. Spinal Accessory

The spinal accessory nerve is not often involved alone. It may be affected by some of the syndromes already mentioned. It is injured in gunshot and stab wounds of the neck, operations on the neck, fracture dislocations of the cervical vertebrae, tumors of the foramen magnum or at the base of the brain, aneurysm, syringomyelia, poliomyelitis, amyotrophic lateral sclerosis, etc. Paralysis of the sternocleidomastoid muscle is characterized by flatness of the neck on the affected side, and failure of the muscle to stand out on rotation of the neck, with decrease of power. The loss of the muscle may be little noticed, the resting posture of the head remaining unchanged. Paralysis of both sternocleidomastoid muscles causes weakness of flexion of the head on the neck. Paralysis of the trapezius muscle causes drooping and inability to raise the shoulder, weakness in shrugging the shoulder, difficulty in raising the arm above the horizontal plane, atrophy and flattening of the neck. The scapula is rotated slightly downward and outward, and in severe instances a slight winging of the scapula occurs.

XII. Hypoglossal

The hypoglossal nerve, like the facial, may show evidence of central or peripheral involvement. Central weakness of the hypoglossal nerve is characterized by deviation of the tongue to the affected side, the tongue being pushed over by the action of the healthy muscles of the opposite side. Such a disturbance is seen in involvement of the tongue fibers at any site from their origin in the opposite motor cortex to its nucleus in the medulla and so is often found in conjunction with hemiplegia, whatever its origin. Rarely it is seen as a single symptom of focal motor cortex disease. It is unassociated with atrophy or muscle fasciculations.

Peripheral weakness is characterized by atrophy of the tongue associated with muscle fasciculations. In early cases the atrophy can be detected as an indentation or scalloping along the edges of the tongue. The detection of atrophy and fasciculations may be difficult early but is of great importance in the differentiation of motor system disease from foramen magnum and cervical cord tumor or

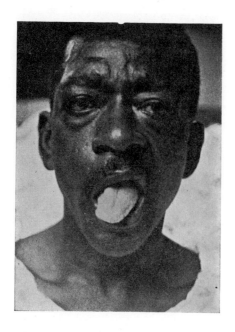

FIGURE 2-19. Lingual paralysis showing the deviation of the tongue to the right side in a case of right hemiplegia.

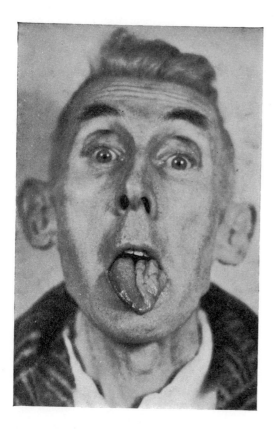

FIGURE 2-20. Hemiatrophy of the tongue in a patient with amyotrophic lateral sclerosis, an instance of nuclear affection.

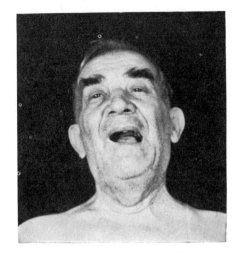

FIGURE 2-21. Lingual paralysis, peripheral in origin, as indicated by the inability to protrude the tongue.

herniated disc. In early cases, fasciculations and atrophy are best studied with the tongue at rest in the floor of the mouth, since stretch of the tongue with protrusion may result in obscuring of both movements and atrophy. As the process becomes more advanced, atrophy becomes more apparent, the tongue shrinking perceptibly on the affected side; with the tongue in the floor of the mouth, a curvature can be seen toward the healthy side. Fasciculations are active when the process is well developed, and the tongue is in a state of lively motion, resembling a "bag of worms." Weakness of the tongue can be demonstrated by pressing the tip of the tongue against the cheek. In severe cases the tongue cannot be protruded. These signs may appear with affection of the nucleus of the hypoglossal nerve in the medulla, as for example in amyotrophic lateral sclerosis, progressive bulbar palsy, syringobulbia, infiltrating tumors, and softening. The nerve may also be involved in both its intramedullary and extramedullary course as is the case with the other lower cranial nerves.

MOTOR SYSTEM

The method of routine examination of the motor system has been indicated in Chapter 1. Examination of the muscles for abnormalities is concerned with a search for disturbance of muscle bulk, power, and tone, involuntary movements, and reflex abnormalities. Evidence of cerebellar dysfunction is also sought.

Muscle Bulk

Changes of *muscle bulk* may manifest themselves either as atrophy or, rarely, hypertrophy. *Atrophy* of muscles is almost always the result of disease of the peripheral pathways, i.e., anterior horn cell, peripheral nerve, or muscle; it may, however, result from cerebral involvement. Its distribution is segmental in the case of anterior horn cell disease or along the distribution of peripheral nerves in case of involvement of these structures. When of cerebral origin it is often associated with an old hemiplegia and may be due to disuse; it may also reflect a trophic disturbance with parietal lobe affection. In infantile hemiplegias both muscles and bones of the affected side are smaller than those of the normal side.

The variety of atrophy occurring with parietal lesions, either softening or tumor, requires special comment. The hand and arm are more affected than the leg. The atrophy of the small hand muscles may simulate closely that of peripheral denervation. The affected muscles are flabby and soft, and the hand is feminine in type. The skin becomes thin and soft, and changes may be seen in the nails.

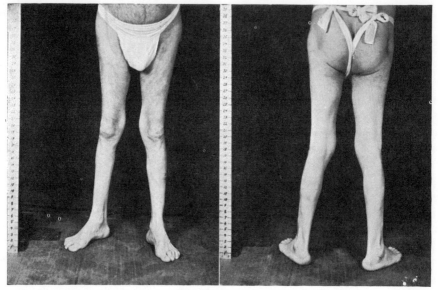

FIGURE 2-22. Atrophy involving the thigh and leg muscles due to poliomyelitis. Note the pes cavus from involvement of the intrinsic foot muscles.

Hemiplegia or hemiparesis is usually but not always present, and varying degrees of sensory impairment may be found. Only position sense of the digits may be affected. The exact reason for the occurrence of this atrophy is unknown; as indicated, it may reflect failure of some trophic influence originating in the parietal lobe.

Segmental atrophy due to cord disease may be difficult to map out because of the innervation of muscles from more than one segment. If the spinal cord disease is not too diffuse, however, it may be possible to determine the segmental character of the atrophy, as in early cases of poliomyelitis with involvement of only a single muscle or a few muscles; or in early cases of amyotrophic lateral sclerosis, syringomyelia, or cervical spondylosis with atrophy of only small hand muscles. The cause of atrophy of denervated muscles due to anterior horn cell disease is not known, but three theories prevail: (1) that it is the result of disuse,

(2) that it is the result of overactivity due to muscle fasciculations (although drugs that increase fibrillary activity have no effect on the rate of atrophy), and (3) that it results from the absence of tension development by denervated muscle.

Muscle atrophy is found in most diseases of the peripheral nerves, regardless of type. The degree and distribution of the atrophy in such instances depend on the extent of the injury of the nerve trunks. Tenderness of the nerve trunks and associated sensory alterations are of assistance in distinguishing the atrophy of peripheral nerve disease from that due to anterior horn cell involvement. Atrophy is found also in cases of arthritis in the muscles contiguous to the affected joints and in muscles that have not been used for some time, as, for example, in muscles encased in a cast. Atrophy is also a characteristic feature of virtually all intrinsic diseases of muscle, i.e., of the myopathies.

There is no constant clinical pattern in the appearance of atrophy after complete or partial denervation. It may develop quickly or slowly and be slight or pronounced. The factors influencing these differences are not known. In anterior horn cell disease the degree of atrophy seems proportional to the number of motor units involved. Presumably the same holds true in peripheral nerve disease. The exact cause of the muscle atrophy in primary muscle disease, as, for example, in the myopathies, is not definitely known.

Muscle *fasciculations* are irregular fine or coarse twitchings of parts of muscles, appearing irregularly and unassociated with movement of the affected muscle at the joint. (*Fibrillations,* which generally appear under much the same circumstances as fasciculations, are usually not visible through the skin, but are recorded electromyographically.) Fasciculations tend to be associated with atrophy of muscles due to denervation and particularly with disease of the anterior horn cells. They are, however, not always seen in atrophied muscle due to advanced anterior horn cell disease because there may be insufficient muscle remaining to exhibit this reaction. Conversely, they may be seen early in anterior horn cell disease with little or no atrophy. They are not, however, present as a rule in acute disease of the anterior horn cells, as in poliomyelitis. Often inconstant, they can be seen in muscles at one time and not at another. At times they are abundant; again they require careful search. They may be brought out on mechanical stimulation of a muscle by tapping or by placing the muscle on stretch. Their exact mode of origin is not known. Though commonly indicative of anterior horn cell disease, fasciculations are seen at times in peripheral nerve disease, particularly when there is associated disease of the anterior roots and anterior horn cells. This occurs especially in the Guillain-Barré syndrome (so-called acute infectious polyradiculoneuropathy) and at times in diabetic or porphyric neuropathy when the entire reflex arc is affected. Fasciculations are also seen in neurotic subjects, in fatigue, on exposure to cold, in thyrotoxicosis, and in a benign condition called *myokymia.* Their predominant occurrence in anterior horn cell disease should nonetheless be emphasized, and when fasciculations are seen, diagnostic consideration should be given to such disorders as progressive spinal muscular atrophy, amyotrophic lateral sclerosis, syringomyelia, infiltrating spinal cord tumor, herniated cervical disc, and other diseases in which the anterior horn cells may be involved.

Muscle *hypertrophy* is found in some forms of myopathy. In pseudo-hypertrophic muscular dystrophy the enlarged muscles have a rubbery consistency, are weak, and are usually associated with atrophy of other muscles. Muscle hypertrophy is found also with prolonged exercise (work hypertrophy); this may occur as a compensatory phenomenon with weakness of other muscles. True muscle hypertrophy is found in association with some forms of congenital disease of the nervous system, in congenital hemihypertrophy involving one half of the body, in hemihypertrophy involving half of the face, and in a very rare disorder involving generalized hypertrophy known as *hypertrophia vera*. It also occurs with myotonia and in cretins.

Muscle Tone

Changes of muscle *tone* must be searched for in any routine examination. There may be increased muscle tone (spasticity or rigidity) or decrease or loss of muscle tone (hypotonia or flaccidity). Interruptions of the corticospinal pathway result in *spasticity,* a condition characterized by an increase in the muscle tone, associated with increase of reflexes, and with pathological reflexes such as the Babinski sign (see Chapter 3). Spastic muscles are associated with an increase of resistance to passive movement followed by a sudden or gradual release of resistance (clasp-knife reaction). The presence of spasticity unfortunately gives no clue as to localization of the lesion producing it. It is indicative only of a lesion causing interruption of the corticospinal pathway anywhere along its course. Thus, spasticity may result from interruption of this pathway in the cerebral hemisphere, in the internal capsule, in the brain stem, or spinal cord. Generally speaking, the farther the lesion from the cortex the more probable is the occurrence of spasticity. Interruption of the corticospinal pathway is, however, by no means invariably associated with spasticity. Particularly in acute cases, decreased muscle tone or flaccidity may follow. Flaccid hemiplegia due to an acutely evolving lesion of the corticospinal system may last a few days to a few weeks or may persist throughout the course of the illness.

There is much doubt as to whether the spasticity of pyramidal lesions is the result of pure corticospinal interruptions or whether it is due to extrapyramidal mechanisms. A variety of clinical and experimental observations indicate that the spasticity and increased reflexes found in corticospinal disease are the result of extrapyramidal, perhaps reticular, rather than pyramidal or corticospinal mechanisms. These extrapyramidal mechanisms apparently act in unopposed fashion under such circumstances, being released from the control of the corticospinal system itself.

Interruption of the extrapyramidal system, on the other hand, results in a state of increased tone referred to as *rigidity*. Rigid muscles reveal a plastic reaction, with an even, steady resistance to passive movement similar to that of bending a lead pipe, hence the term "lead-pipe rigidity" given to this form of increased tonus. At times, the rigidity may be intermittent and jerky, as in the "cogwheel" rigidity of parkinsonism.

Hypotonia or *flaccidity* is characteristic of peripheral involvement and is invariably associated with disease of the anterior horn cells and peripheral nerves. The muscles are toneless, loose, their normal rounded contour is replaced by a flattened appearance, and the affected limbs are hyperextended at the joints and flail-like in their looseness. Hypotonia may be encountered with disease of the posterior roots, presumably as a result of interruption of the intrafusal fibers within the afferent limb of the reflex arcs ordinarily operative in the maintenance of normal tone. Hypotonia is found also in cerebellar lesions; it is more likely to be associated with acute injuries or disease of the cerebellum than with chronic conditions. Some degree of hypotonia may be observed, at least in the experimental animal, with lesions in the posterior columns of the spinal cord as well.

Muscle Power

Changes of muscle *power* are invariably associated with disease either of the upper or lower motor neuron or of the muscles. The degree of weakness depends on the degree of injury of the anterior horn cells, peripheral nerves, motor pathways, muscles, or other motor units anywhere in the neuraxis. The weakness may be partial, in which case it is referred to as *paresis,* or it may be complete when it is of course designated as *paralysis.* The weakness of anterior horn cell disease is segmental in character and associated with flaccidity, atrophy, fasciculations, and loss of reflexes. That of peripheral nerve disease follows the distribution of the affected nerve or nerves and is thus predominantly distal in the common polyneuropathies; it is often associated with pain and sensory disturbances and is accompanied by loss of reflexes. Weakness of upper motor neuron disease is hemiplegic in character, usually affects distal more than proximal muscles, is associated with spasticity, overactive reflexes, and pathological reflexes, and is without sensory changes. Apparent weakness is found in diseases of the extrapyramidal system; however, it is the result not of true weakness, but of slowness in initiating movement.

Not all weakness results directly from disease of the central or peripheral nervous system. Primary diseases of muscles (myopathies) are invariably associated with weakness, almost always proximal in distribution. Marked weakness results from interference with neuromuscular transmission as in myasthenia gravis, curare poisoning, and botulism. Transient paralysis occurs in such electrolyte disorders as severe hypokalemia and is characteristic of the periodic paralyses related to serum potassium levels; in these instances interference with transmission of the electrotonic impulse along the sarcolemmal membrane is possibly the factor responsible for weakness.

Attacks of generalized muscular weakness, induced by emotional excitement of any sort and resulting in complete transitory collapse, are found in the *cataplectic* attacks of *narcolepsy,* although here the mechanism of production is unknown. A number of patients so afflicted also wake from sleep on occasion to find themselves virtually completely paralyzed for greater or lesser periods (so-called *sleep paralysis*).

Loss of movement, it should be emphasized, is by no means necessarily indicative of paralysis per se, a simple fact that is sometimes overlooked. Profound impairment of movement often occurs with severe *sensory deprivation,* particularly of proprioception, without actual dysfunction of the motor apparatus itself; in cases such as these the apparent weakness improves remarkably if the patient watches the limb during attempted movement. Loss or decrease of movement is seen characteristically in paralysis agitans, unassociated with weakness of any degree. This is seen in early cases as a loss of the normal arm swing and later as loss of almost all voluntary movement. Loss of movement may result from contractures or from fixation of joints by trophic or other processes. It may be associated also with catatonia and with hysteria, the latter without organic changes of any sort.

Accessory or *associated* or *synkinetic* movements are seen under some circumstances, especially in disease of the corticospinal system. Flexion movements of the fingers of the paralyzed hand may be observed in cases of hemiplegia when a patient squeezes the examiner's hand with the normal hand, and dorsiflexion of the paralyzed foot often occurs on flexion of the paretic leg. Dorsiflexion of the paretic foot in hemiplegia is seen on flexion of the knee (*Strümpell phenomenon*); pronation of the paretic forearm is found on extension of both arms upward (pronator sign). In *Hoover's sign,* with the hands held under the patient's heels while he is on his back, lifting the paralyzed leg results in an increased downward pressure with the sound leg. This is valuable in differentiating a hemiplegia of organic or structural origin from one of hysterical origin since the downward pressure of the normal leg will be absent in the hysterical patient.

Involuntary Movements

Involuntary muscular movements occur in a variety of forms and under many circumstances. Fasciculations and myokymia have been described above. Other patterns of movement disorders are as follows:

TREMOR. Defined as involuntary, purposeless, and generally rhythmical movements of the limbs, and, on occasion, of the head and trunk, tremor may be most simply approached on the basis of the circumstances under which the movements appear.

A tremor that is present when the limbs are in complete repose is referred to as a *resting tremor* and is characteristically encountered in instances of paralysis agitans (parkinsonism). The tremor is quite rapid, affects particularly the distal muscles (forearms and hands), and often assumes a pill-rolling quality. It may persist, sometimes with increase in amplitude when the arms are held extended, but with volitional movement customarily diminishes, returning to its prior severity when the limb again rests. A rather similar resting tremor may be encountered in hepatolenticular degeneration (Wilson's disease). In that condition, a much more florid movement disorder appears when the arms are held abducted, consisting of coarse irregular flapping movements referred to as a *wing-beating tremor.* A similar but usually much finer flapping tremor may be encountered in the metabolic encephalopathies found in liver or pulmonary disease and tends to be quite prominent in cases of impending hepatic coma. The term *asterixis* is sometimes applied to a tremor of this sort.

In many conditions, tremor appears only when the arms are held extended. Thus, a fine and rapid tremor of the outstretched fingers is found in general paresis, commonly associated with tremors of the tongue, eyelids, and lips. Fine tremors of the fingers also appear in thyrotoxicosis, in conditions of fatigue or excitement, after the administration of such agents as epinephrine, amphetamine, or ephedrine, and in anxiety neurosis. The use of cocaine, barbiturates, morphine, and bromides is often attended by similar movements, and tremors of this sort may follow exposure to such industrial toxins as mercury. Coarse tremors of the outstretched fingers commonly appear in the chronic alcoholic and can be very severe during withdrawal from alcohol, as in the states of alcoholic tremulousness and delirium tremens; a curious inner sense of tremulousness often accompanies the somatic tremors under these circumstances.

A coarse tremor of the outstretched fingers, sometimes increasing with voluntary activity, is the so-called *familial tremor*. This tends to appear chiefly in males, the onset of movement being at times as early as adolescence. The same type of slowly progressive tremor may appear later in life, without a positive family history; under these circumstances the term *benign essential tremor* is used. In both varieties, it tends to begin in the arms and may lead to considerable embarrassment as a result of spillage of food and drink. Eventually tremor of the head may appear, and the voice characteristically becomes quavering. The movements are suppressed by alcohol, and this may lead to excessive utilization with chronic alcoholism as a result. These conditions are often mistakenly diagnosed as paralysis agitans even though unassociated with other signs of extrapyramidal disease.

Coarse tremor of the fingers, generally in conjunction with either a nodding or rotary tremor of the head, is found in late life and is referred to as *senile tremor*. The movements may be found at rest, on movement, or with extension. A tremor of the tongue may also be present. Ordinarily there are no signs to suggest the presence of significant extrapyramidal disease.

Tremor, or more accurately tremulousness, may appear in a paretic limb during attempted movement. This is a nonrhythmical movement, generally more proximal than distal, and is probably due to faulty postural fixation of the limb concerned.

Disease of the cerebellum or its pathways results in the appearance of an *intention tremor,* characterized by the development of oscillating fairly regular movements on voluntary movement, of increasing amplitude as the goal is approached. Usually no tremor is evident at rest, but some movements may be visible when the arms are simply held extended. Intention tremor appears most prominently with involvement of the superior cerebellar peduncle (brachium conjunctivum); it thus appears most strikingly with softenings following occlusion of the superior cerebellar artery or with any other lesion implicating the dentato-rubral pathway, as, for example, in multiple sclerosis.

CHOREA. Choreic movements are quick movements of rather small amplitude, sometimes explosive in occurrence, involving both distal and proximal muscles;

most frequently the hands are affected, and a constant play of twitching movements of the fingers may be seen. Chorea is generally associated with some degree of hypotonia of muscles. It characteristically occurs in Sydenham's (rheumatic) chorea, chorea gravidarum, and Huntington's chorea, but similar movements are occasionally seen under other circumstances as well. The movements of chorea may be very gross, capable of moving an entire limb in an irregular, abrupt, flinging fashion (hemichorea); it may be very difficult to distinguish this from *hemiballismus,* a dramatic condition characterized by wild flinging or circling movements of the limbs, tending to involve the arm more than the leg, and most commonly associated with focal lesions of the subthalamic nucleus.

ATHETOSIS. In contrast to the abrupt and predominantly distal movements of chorea, athetosis is characterized by slower snakelike movements, involving distal muscles but with a tendency to spread proximally as well. Muscle tone is somewhat heightened as a rule. This may appear in many disorders affecting the basal ganglia, as, for example, softenings and infections. It is also found in so-called double athetosis, a condition of infancy and childhood possibly reflecting birth hypoxia and associated pathologically with status marmoratus (marbled state, "hypermyelinization") of the basal nuclear masses. Athetotic-like movements are seen in a variety of diseases characterized by a loss of proprioception in the involved limbs, such as subacute combined degeneration of the cord and tabes dorsalis; it also appears not uncommonly during recovery from hemiplegia (*posthemiplegic athetosis* or *chorea*), and under these circumstances impairment of proprioception is also found.

DYSTONIA. This consists of slow writhing movements, sometimes beginning in the distal portions of the limbs but spreading proximally to involve the proximal muscles and the head, neck, and trunk, reaching its most florid manifestation in that disease known as *dystonia musculorum deformans.* As with chorea and athetosis, dystonia tends to be related primarily to basal ganglia dysfunction. In terms of speed of movement, distribution of movement, and muscle tone, it stands at the opposite end of the scale from chorea, with athetosis between.

MYOCLONUS. Myoclonic movements are rapid contractions of either proximal or distal muscles, usually nonrhythmic but sometimes bilaterally symmetrical, and found in many conditions. They are seen in disorders characterized by extensive destruction of cortical neurons, such as Tay-Sachs disease and Jakob-Creutzfeldt disease, as well as in inclusion body encephalitis, which is characterized by damage to both gray and white matter of the cerebrum. They are an important feature of so-called myoclonus epilepsy of Unverricht, in which major changes may be present in the cerebellar cortex or deep nuclei. In a rare infantile disease known as infantile spasms, associated with remarkable electroencephalographic changes called hypsarhythmia, massive myoclonic jerks of the trunk are prominent. Rapid fluttering rhythmical movements of the soft palate, sometimes with synchronous movements of the eyes, tongue, and jaw, are referred to as *palatal myoclonus* (or *palatal nystagmus*); this results from interruption of the dentato-rubro-olivary neural system, usually by softening.

SPASMS. Spasms of various kinds are seen in nervous disorders. Habit spasms of many sorts are common, involving face, limbs, or trunk. Spasmodic torticollis is a variety of spasm involving the neck muscles, resulting in movement of the head, and may represent a limited variety of dystonic movements. Hemispasm of the face, associated with lesions of the facial nerve, or occurring as a habit spasm, is sometimes seen. Blepharospasms are found following encephalitis and consist of spasmodic contractions of the eyelids. Spasms of the tongue and spasms of swallowing are seen at times, the former in states of emotional instability, or in conjunction with reflex irritation from throat, teeth, or mouth infections, and the latter in neuroses.

CONVULSIONS. These vary greatly as to type, cause, and expression, and careful observation of their clinical features may give valuable information as to the locus of the responsible epileptogenic focus. A detailed discussion of the subject is not, however, within the scope of this presentation.

Reflex Disturbances

The common reflexes that should be examined routinely have been referred to in Chapter 1.

LOSS OF TENDON REFLEXES. This occurs most frequently in cases of interruption of the reflex arc, whether it be in anterior horns, anterior roots, peripheral nerve, or posterior roots. The features that distinguish interruption of the reflex arc at its various levels are described in Chapter 3. Loss of reflexes may occur also in the myopathies, usually in advanced stages of the disease and associated with muscle atrophy. The reflexes are lost temporarily during the periods of paralysis of familial periodic paralysis. In instances of spinal shock in which there has been acute transection or acute compression of the cord, flaccid paralysis and loss of reflexes are characteristic. The stage of spinal shock may persist for 2 weeks to 2 or 3 months and be replaced by spasticity and overactive reflexes, or it may persist indefinitely. The tendon reflexes may also disappear in instances of overwhelming sepsis. Rarely, in normal subjects no patellar reflexes may be elicited or there may be loss of all tendon reflexes.

INCREASE OR EXAGGERATION OF TENDON REFLEXES. These occur in the vast majority of instances as a result of disease of the corticospinal pathways. In such instances, the exaggerated reflexes are associated with abnormal reflexes such as the extensor plantar. Overactive reflexes are sometimes but not consistently found in extrapyramidal diseases such as paralysis agitans. Increase of reflexes is seen often in neurotic subjects but not accompanied by pathological responses.

ABNORMAL REFLEXES. *Babinski Sign.* Associated with increased reflexes are various abnormal reflexes seen in disease of the corticospinal system. Chief among these reflexes is the Babinski toe sign, consisting of extension of the great toe, usually with spreading and flexion of the small toes, on stroking the outer edge of the sole of the foot. It is probably better to refer to this sign as the *extensor plantar response,* since Babinski's name is actually applied to a number of other physical signs; traditionally, however, the term Babinski's sign is applied to this reflex above all. This sign is pathognomonic of corticospinal disease. It is never present in normal subjects except in infants during the first 6 months of life. While a Babinski sign always indicates disease of the corticospinal pathway, it is not invariably present under such circumstances, although other evidence of disease of this system may be abundant. Conversely, the Babinski sign may be the only evidence of corticospinal disease or the only residual of previous and more extensive disease. Care must be taken to avoid interpretation of a voluntary withdrawal extensor toe response as a Babinski sign. The toe extension in cortico-spinal disease is slow and usually disappears soon after the stimulus is removed; that of a voluntary response is faster and associated with rapid withdrawal of the leg. Transient extensor plantar responses may be found following generalized convulsions, in coma, and in many diffuse encephalopathies.

None of the other signs that have been described in corticospinal tract disease appears with the same constancy as the Babinski sign.

Oppenheim's Sign. Extension of the great toe on firm downward stroking along the medial side of the tibia is indicative of corticospinal disease but is not constant.

Chaddock's Sign. This consists of extension of the great toe on stroking the dorsum of the foot on its outer edge in the presence of corticospinal disease.

Gordon's Sign. Extension of the toe on firm compression of the calf; it too appears in corticospinal disease.

Rossolimo's Sign. It consists of plantar flexion of the toes on tapping the balls of the toes. This sign is an unreliable indicator of pyramidal disease when found alone without a Babinski sign or evidence of weakness. It is normally found in children from 2 to 3 months to 2 to 3 years of age. A similar flexion of the toes is seen in *Mendel-Bechterew's sign,* elicited by tapping the dorsum of the foot on its outer surface over the cuboid bone; it is much less common than the Rossolimo sign.

Table 2-1. Pathological Reflexes of Lower Extremity

Reflex	Stimulus	Response
BABINSKI	Stroking outer edge of sole of foot	1. Extension of great toe 2. Flexion of small toes 3. Spreading of small toes 4. Flexion of leg
CHADDOCK	Stroking lateral aspect of dorsum of foot and external malleolus	Extension of great toe
OPPENHEIM	Firm downward stroking of medial aspect of tibia	Extension of great toe
ROSSOLIMO	Tapping balls of toes	Plantar flexion of toes
MENDEL-BECHTEREW	Tapping dorsum of foot on outer surface	Plantar flexion of toes

Hoffmann's Sign. In the upper extremity the Hoffmann sign is said to be indicative of corticospinal disease, but it probably indicates only a state of heightened reflex activity. It is elicited by lightly flicking the terminal phalanx of the middle finger, or by snapping the nail of the middle finger, the resulting response being a flexion and adduction movement of the thumb and flexion of the fingers.

Trömner's Reflex. This is a modification of the finger flexor reflex and is elicited as follows: The patient keeps his fingers flexed while the examiner taps with his middle finger the palmar surface of the tip of the middle or index finger of the patient. A positive response is indicated by flexion of all the fingers including the thumb. As with the Hoffmann, this was regarded erroneously as indicative of corticospinal disease, but implies only increased muscle tone of the fingers.

Finger-Thumb Reflex (Mayer). This reflex consists of opposition and adduction of the thumb combined with flexion at the metacarpophalangeal joint on firm passive flexion of the third to the fifth finger at the proximal joints. The reflex is positive in normal persons and absent in patients with corticospinal lesions. When lost on one side it may constitute an important sign of a pyramidal tract lesion.

Withdrawal (Flexor) Reflexes of Spinal Automatism. After transection of the spinal cord, a state of spinal shock develops during which all reflex activity below the level of the lesion is lost. As recovery ensues, segmental reflex activity returns and is seen first in a return of the flexion reflexes of the toes and feet, followed in the course of time by flexion of the entire lower extremity.

Flexion reflexes in transecting lesions of the spinal cord are elicited by stimulating the skin of the trunk or limbs below the level of the lesion by pinching, pin prick, scratching, application of cold, stroking the sole of the foot, or by the use of any noxious stimulus. The result is a massive reflex movement of flexion of the thighs and legs with dorsiflexion of the foot and toes. The movement is sometimes mistaken by the patient for a voluntary movement and as an indication of improvement.

Such reflexes are seen most commonly in instances of complete interruption of the spinal cord by transection due to injury, compression, vascular disease, etc. They also appear, however, without complete transection, in the presence of bilateral pyramidal tract disease, as in spastic paraplegias. The Babinski sign itself may be regarded as a fraction of a flexion reflex. In spastic paraplegia, stimulation of one leg will often result in flexion of this leg with crossed extension of the opposite limb. This is known as *Philippson's reflex.* In spinal man, that is, in a subject in whom the spinal cord has been transected from some cause, there ensues on scratching or stimulating any part of the legs a *mass reflex* characterized by flexor spasm of the ventral abdominal wall and lower extremities, evacuation of the bladder, and sweating from an area of skin varying with the level of the lesion.

Postural Reflexes. These are much more evident in experimental situations than in clinical practice. In decerebrate animals destruction of the labyrinths permits full exploration of the *tonic neck reflexes.* Thus, rotation of the head causes an increase in extensor tonus of the limb toward which the jaw points ("jaw limb") and relaxation of the limb toward which the vertex is rotated ("skull limb"). Furthermore, flexion of the head toward one shoulder causes extension of the jaw

Table 2-2. Pathological Hand Reflexes Resulting from Lesions of the Pyramidal Tract

Name	Stimulus	Response
PALM-CHIN REFLEX (*Marinesco-Radiovici*)	Stimulation of hyperthenar region (ulnar, median)	Contraction of muscles of chin and elevation of corner of mouth
THUMB-ADDUCTOR REFLEX (*"Babinski of the hand"*) MARIE-FOIX OF THE HAND	Superficial stroking of hypothenar region (ulnar)	Adduction and flexion of thumb; sometimes flexion of adjacent digits and extension of little finger
EXTENSION-ADDUCTION REFLEX (*Dagnini*)	Percussion of dorsum of hand (radial)	Slight adduction and extension of wrist
"MENDEL-BECHTEREW OF THE HAND"	Percussion of dorsal aspect of carpus and metacarpus (radial)	Flexion of fingers
"ROSSOLIMO OF THE HAND"	Percussion of palmar aspect of metacarpophalangeal joint	Flexion of fingers
HOFFMANN'S SIGN	Snapping nail of middle finger (median)	Flexion of thumb and fingers
TRÖMNER'S SIGN	Tapping palmar surface of tip of middle or index finger	Flexion of fingers and thumb
GORDON'S SIGN	Compression of region of pisiform bone (ulnar)	Extension of flexed fingers
CHADDOCK'S SIGN	Pressure of tendon of palmaris longus muscle	Flexion of wrist; extension of fingers

Synkinesis of Upper Extremity in Cases of Pyramidal Lesions

Name	Stimulus	Response
WARTENBERG'S SIGN	Active flexion of fingers about a stick	Flexion and opposition of thumb
SIGN OF KLIPPEL AND WEIL	Passive extension of fingers (when there is some contracture in flexion)	Flexion and opposition of thumb
SOUQUES' SIGN OF INTEROSSEOUS MUSCLES	Active elevation of extended arm	Extension and adduction of fingers
STRÜMPELL'S SIGN	Active flexion of elbow	Pronation and flexion of hand
BRACHIOBRACHIAL SYNKINESIS	Extension of flexed elbow of normal side by examiner, against patient's resistance	Flexion of elbow on paralyzed side
STERLING'S SIGN	Active adduction of shoulder on normal side against resistance by examiner	Adduction of shoulder on paretic side

limbs and relaxation of the skull limbs; extension of the head causes extension of the forelimbs and flexion of the hind limbs; and flexion of the head causes flexion of the forelimbs and extension of the hind limbs. Counterparts of these reflexes are seen in some conditions in the human, particularly in infants up to 12 weeks of age, and in some cases of brain stem or bilateral corticospinal disease. A special neck reflex occurring in infants has been described by Landau. If an infant during the second year is supported under the chest by one hand, the neck extends, the back arches, and the extremities extend. If the head is passively flexed in such a case the extension of trunk and limb vanishes and the baby folds up like a jackknife. Another special reflex is the *Moro reflex,* in which all four extremities are thrown into sudden rigid extension if the supporting surface on which the infant lies is suddenly jarred or shaken. It is present in infants for about the first 3 months of life.

Tonic *labyrinthine reflexes* can be studied in decerebrate animals by section of the cervical roots, thus eliminating the neck reflexes. Under such conditions it can be demonstrated that marked changes occur in posture and muscle tonus with variation of the body in space, maximal extension occurring in the supine position with the snout about 45 degrees above the horizontal plane and minimal extension with the snout 45 degrees below the horizontal. The reflexes are dependent upon intact labyrinths, taking their origin in the otoliths, and disappear completely after bilateral labyrinthectomy. These reflexes are undoubtedly of importance in the human but are of little significance in clinical diagnosis. The same may be said of the *righting reflexes,* which are the mechanisms whereby the animal attempts to bring body and head into normal position by means of labyrinthine, neck, optical, body-to-head, and body-to-body reflexes.

Of greater clinical significance is the *grasp reflex* that is found in paretic limbs. It is characterized by grasping movements in response to objects seen or contacts felt in the palm of the hand, and reflex tonic grasping in response to stretching the flexor muscles of the fingers. The greater the stretch, the stronger the grasp. The grasp reflex is unaffected by loss of sensation of the skin of the hand and by visual stimuli since it is found with undiminished intensity after local anesthesia of the hand and after blindfolding. It is present without hypertonicity of the muscles. It is regarded by most observers as a purely reflex phenomenon, but some believe a volitional element is present. In the experimental animal it is influenced by righting, neck, and labyrinthine reflex mechanisms.

The grasp reflex and forced grasping have been found to indicate in humans lesions of the opposite frontal lobe but are normal phenomena in infants. The opposite of grasping, i.e., *avoidance,* is sometimes encountered with parietal lesions.

The *superficial reflexes* are disturbed in many conditions. The *abdominal reflexes* are lost in hemiplegia on the side of the pyramidal tract dysfunction, as are the *cremasteric reflexes;* this is not invariable, however. The *corneal reflex,* when lost, is a sign of great significance. It may be absent as the result of local disease of the cornea. It is always absent or decreased in cases of fresh hemiplegia, and it is absent in lesions that involve the sensory trigeminal nucleus in the pons and in lesions of the trigeminal root or ganglion. It is often lost early in cerebellopontine angle tumors.

Additional Reflexes. The *orbicularis oculi reflex* is elicited as follows: The skin at the outer corner of the eye is held between the thumb and index finger, pulling it back slightly, and the thumb is tapped lightly with a reflex hammer. There follows a reflex contraction of the orbicularis oculi muscle. Diminution of the reflex is found in facial palsies of peripheral origin. It is preserved in central facial palsies. The response obtained is a deep muscle reflex. The *jaw reflex* is elicited by tapping the mandible with the jaw half opened, the lower jaw moving briskly upward. It is increased in bilateral supranuclear cerebral lesions. The *snout reflex* is brought out by tapping in the midline of maxilla or mandible and consists of a rooting movement of the lips; it is found in instances of diffuse cerebral dysfunction. The *sucking reflex* consists of involuntary pursing of the lips in response to visual or tactile stimuli. It is normal in infants but appears in later life as a sign, either unilateral or bilateral, of frontal or diffuse cerebral damage. Like the grasp, it represents a return to a more primitive level of function.

The *scapulohumeral reflex* is elicited by tapping the vertebral border of the scapula with resulting contraction of muscles of the shoulder girdle and arm. Many muscles are brought into play, especially the deltoids, pectoralis major, infraspinatus, and teres minor. Adduction of the arm occurs. Unilateral absence of the reflex is found in lesions of the fifth cervical segment. The *adductor reflex of the thigh* is obtained by placing the finger on the medial condyle of the femur with the leg slightly abducted. When the finger is tapped adduction of the leg follows. The *biceps femoris reflex* is best elicited with the patient lying on the side opposite the one being examined, the leg being bent at the hip and knee. The finger is placed on the hamstring tendon and is tapped with a reflex hammer. Contraction of the muscle results. The *scapular reflex*, elicited by stroking the skin between the scapulae, results in contraction of the scapular muscles. The *gluteal reflex* results in contraction of the glutei on stroking the skin of the buttock.

Disturbances of Station

Standing is a postural reflex dependent on reflexes mediated through the medulla oblongata and influenced to a marked degree by tonic neck, labyrinthine, cerebellar and proprioceptive mechanisms. Interference with any of the mechanisms responsible for the maintenance of local, segmental, or general static postural reflexes will cause impairment of the act of normal standing. Weakness or deformity of the legs will, of course, also interfere with the stance, though on an entirely different basis.

Disturbances of station are characterized primarily by inability to maintain normal equilibrium in standing, with the eyes either open or closed. As found in disease of the posterior roots or columns (tabes dorsalis, subacute combined degeneration, Friedreich's ataxia, etc.), the difficulty is dependent on loss or impairment of deep sensation, manifested by a loss of position sense in the joints. Under these circumstances, *Romberg's sign* is positive; this is characterized classically by inability to stand steadily with the feet together, the difficulty being increased with the eyes closed. A Romberg sign may be regarded as positive only if there is actual loss of balance during the maneuver, with a shift in the position of the feet in order to maintain equilibrium. Swaying of the trunk without loss of equilibrium cannot be regarded as a positive Romberg sign.

If in early or mild cases Romberg's sign is not convincing, more definite difficulties may be brought out by asking the patient to maintain his balance on one leg alone with the eyes open or closed. This is well done by normal subjects but difficult or impossible for the patient with even mild disease of the posterior columns.

Disturbances of station are also found in diseases of the cerebellum or its pathways. In cases of cerebellar disease associated with truncal incoordination there is inability to stand with the feet close together with the eyes either open or closed. Indeed, standing unsupported becomes impossible in advanced cases even with the legs widely separated. It should be emphasized that the disability in cerebellar disease, unlike that of posterior column disease, is not seriously affected by closing the eyes and is not dependent on loss of deep sensation.

Interference with standing is found in disease of the labyrinths, the vestibular pathways, or in any disorder in which vertigo is prominent; in such instances it results from interference with spatial orientation and the false sense of motion associated with the sensation of vertigo. Patients with dizziness are unable to stand even with the legs widely separated, and they cannot walk a straight course.

Disturbances of Gait

Impairment or loss of the normal act of walking is encountered in a wide variety of neurological diseases. The act of normal locomotion is influenced by a number of bodily mechanisms and is the result of integration of many types of reflexes. It is dependent on simple reflex mechanisms at the spinal cord level, on righting reflexes maintaining the proper position of head, limbs, and trunk against gravity, on postural reflexes holding the body erect by maintaining extensor tone, and on neck and labyrinthine reflexes for regulating muscle tone, and providing proper spatial orientation. It is also, of course, dependent upon normal strength and sensibility. Under these circumstances, walking may be abnormal as the result of such diverse factors as disintegration of spinal cord reflex mechanisms, brain stem disorders, vestibular and cerebellar disturbances, proprioceptive loss, pyramidal tract disease, and cortical disintegration.

STEPPAGE GAIT. Primarily a peripheral variety of gait alteration, the steppage gait is associated with foot drop and is seen in simplest form with a lesion of the external popliteal nerve itself or in its innervation from spinal cord segments L5-S1. The leg is flaccid and the gait characterized by foot drop, with marked elevation of the thigh and leg in order to clear the dropped foot from the ground. The condition is sometimes bilateral, as, for example, with tumors involving the cauda equina or in bilateral involvement of the spinal cord segments in poliomyelitis. It is also bilateral in cases of peroneal muscular atrophy (Charcot-Marie-Tooth disease), and in advanced polyneuropathies of diverse cause.

Unilateral foot drop may be seen in sciatic neuritis or in sciatica due to herniated intervertebral disc. Another form of gait disorder may also be seen in cases of sciatica. In such instances, the knee and hip are flexed on the painful side, the pelvis drops toward the painful side, and the gait is carried out with short steps, the limb being flexed to avoid stretching the sciatic nerve.

A peculiar gait, also of peripheral origin and due to pain, is that seen in cases of peripheral neuropathy (particularly of the "alcoholic" nutritional variety), in causalgias due to nerve injuries, or in vasomotor disorders (erythromelalgia), all associated with painful hyperesthesias of the soles of the foot. In such cases weight bearing is painful. The gait is with short steps, and limping and halting in character. The feet are commonly rotated in such a position as to avoid walking on the painful portions.

WADDLING GAIT.   This is seen in cases of muscular dystrophy and other varieties of proximal muscular affection and is characterized by a wide base, lordosis, and a peculiar waddle with extension and lateral movement of the pelvis due to weakness of the gluteal and truncal muscles.

HYPOTONIC (TABETIC) GAIT.   This gait abnormality, with hyperextension of the knees and loose, flail-like joints, is seen most characteristically in tabes dorsalis. The gait is broad based in order to shift the center of gravity, with the legs lifted high in walking, slapped down firmly on the ground in order to elicit what proprioceptive reflexes may be available, and with the eyes carefully watching the feet. The abnormality is greatly increased in the dark and with the eyes closed. Similar types of gait are found in any disease of the posterior columns. At least superficially, this disability resembles the ataxic gait of cerebellar disease.

CEREBELLAR (ATAXIC) GAIT.   This is characterized by inability of truncal, pelvic, and limb muscles to move in unison in a coordinated fashion. The patient walks with a widened base, the pelvis held stiffly and tilted somewhat anteriorly, the trunk and limbs seemingly independent of the pelvis. The result is a disorganized gait with marked ataxia, the legs thrust forward from the hip in mechanical fashion without direction or coordination. Lurching and staggering are common. So incoordinate is the performance that patients with cerebellar disease are often accused of intoxication. Patients with this sort of gait abnormality generally have a lesion of the midline of the cerebellum, i.e., the vermis. The head may be held stiffly and anteriorly flexed, particularly in cases of midline cerebellar tumors and in those that obstruct the fourth ventricle. A staggering, reeling ataxic gait is also encountered during acute vestibular disease, as in labyrinthitis, or in interruption of the vestibular pathways in the brain stem. Under such circumstances, the patient generally complains of *vertigo,* and associated signs of vestibular disease are found.

SPASTIC GAIT.   Disease of the corticospinal system is associated with gait disorders characterized primarily by spasticity. Chief among these is the *hemiplegic gait,* in which the arm is held spastically in a semiflexed adducted posture and the leg spastic, extended, circumducted, and plantar flexed, a pattern so characteristic that it can hardly be misinterpreted. Bilateral disease of the corticospinal pathways results in a *spastic gait,* a shuffling type of gait with the legs stiff, extended, and scraping over the surface without being lifted from the ground. In some types of spastic gait the legs, spastic while attempting to walk, are quite limber on recumbency. In cerebral diplegia the severe spasticity of the legs results in a *scissors gait,* in which the legs cross over in front of one another as each is put forward, resulting in a scissors-like action; spasticity here is usually very severe, and associated with pronounced adductor hypertonicity.

BASAL GANGLIA GAIT DISORDERS. Abnormalities of gait are seen in basal ganglia disorders, especially in *paralysis agitans.* In early cases only a loss of automatic swinging of the arms is seen while walking; in advanced cases the head and body are flexed, the arms semiflexed and adducted in a posture reminiscent of a spastic attitude, the legs flexed and rigid, and the gait slow and shuffling (*marche à petits pas; festination*). Initiation of the act of walking is slow, so that there may be a long latency between arising from a chair and the beginning of the walking act. The gait is often propulsive, the patient walking with increasing rapidity as if chasing his own center of gravity; at times the reverse, i.e., a retropulsive gait, is seen. In *dystonia musculorum deformans* severe contortions give a ludicrous, bizarre appearance to the gait. In the various illness in which *chorea* is found, the sudden movements of the limbs or trunk may interfere with walking, at least in fleeting fashion.

HYSTERICAL GAIT. Not easily described, the principal feature of a hysterical gait is the bizarre character; any sort of performance may be encountered. *Astasia-abasia,* or complete inability to stand or walk, may be seen in hysteria. It may also be encountered, however, with bilateral cerebral (particularly frontoparietal) disease as an expression of *gait apraxia.*

A short-stepped, shuffling gait similar to that of parkinsonism may also be encountered in senile individuals and those with extensive cerebrovascular disease.

Disturbances of Coordination

The smooth coordination of muscular movement is impaired or lost under many different circumstances in diseases of the nervous system. Since normal coordination depends upon the proper functioning of agonists, antagonists, and synergists, it follows that any interference with the normal interrelationships of these muscle groups will result in incoordination. *Weakness* of a muscle or limb will thus cause loss of coordination of movement because of muscular imbalance. A paretic arm consequently exhibits difficulty in performing smoothly the finger-nose test or rapid pronation and supination. Incoordination is also seen in the impairment of the finer movements of the thumb and fingers, particularly the index finger, in cases of disease of the corticospinal pathways. Fine movements, such as buttoning clothes and picking up small objects, are often lost.

Incoordination is found in instances of interruption of the *posterior columns,* or its brain stem prolongation, the mesial fillet. Under these circumstances, the incoordination, or *ataxia* as it may be called, is dependent on loss of proprioceptive impulses, is accompanied by loss of position or vibration sense, or both, and is increased on closing the eyes. The ataxia of posterior column disease is characterized by *dysmetria,* that is, errors in range of movement. There is inability to measure distance properly, and overshooting of the goal results. Tremor may accompany the movement.

Table 2-3. Differentiation of Cerebellar and Posterior Column Incoordination

	Cerebellar	*Posterior Column*
SENSORY DISTURBANCES	Absent	Always present Loss or impairment of position and vibration senses
VISION	Symptoms not increased by shutting out vision	Symptoms increased by obliteration of vision
DYSMETRIA	Reaches goal with tremor, or overshoots and finally settles on it	Overshoots goal and fails to find it with eyes closed
TREMOR	On voluntary movement	Incoordination tremor
GAIT	Wide-based, pelvis fixed, trunk and limbs moving asynchronously	Wide-based, steppage with eyes watching feet and ground
STATION	Romberg's sign not present, but unsteadiness in standing with eyes open or closed	Romberg's sign present

A special form of incoordination known as *asynergia* or *dyssynergia* is found in cerebellar disease. This is not dependent on disturbances of sensation. It is characterized by dysmetria, inability to perform movements smoothly (pronation-supination movements of the arms, rapid patting with the hands), and by disturbance of gait. Cerebellar dyssynergia may be mild or severe and may involve any or all parts of the body. Slight degrees of dyssynergia are brought out by the pronation-supination test; the patient is clumsy, the arm swings out more than normally, he overpronates or supinates and loses the beat of the rhythmic movement of the test. In severe cases no rhythmic movement is possible. The cerebellar gait, which may be looked upon as an expression of the dyssynergia of the trunk muscles, has already been described. It should be pointed out that the basic defect in all manifestation of incoordination in cerebellar disease may be one of faulty postural fixation, particularly at proximal joints.

Disease of the *labyrinths,* the vestibular nerve, and the vestibular pathways in the brain stem is also associated with incoordination characterized particularly by dysmetria, with past pointing. The presence of nystagmus and most especially of vertigo may assist in separating this from the deficit encountered in cerebellar disease.

SENSATION

The methods of performing a sensory examination have been described in Chapter 1. The various patterns of altered sensibility consequent to lesions at the peripheral, radicular, spinal cord, brain stem, thalamic, and cortical levels will be discussed in Chapter 3.

BIBLIOGRAPHY

Adie, W. J.: Tonic Pupils and Absent Tendon Reflexes. Brain 55:98, 1932.

Alpers, B. J., and Forster, F. M.: Site and Origin of Fasciculations in Voluntary Muscle. Arch. Neurol. Psychiat. 51:264, 1944.

Alpers, B. J., Forster, F. M., and Borkowski, W. J.: Effects of Denervation on Fasciculations in Human Muscle. Arch. Neurol. Psychiat. 56:276, 1946.

Barré, J. A.: Le syndrome pyramidal déficitaire. Rev. neurol. 67:1, 1937.

Bender, M. B., and Strauss, I.: Defects in Visual Fields of One Eye Only in Patients with a Lesion of One Optic Radiation. Arch. Ophthal. 17:765, 1937.

Bennett, H. S., Szent-Gyorgyi, A., Denny-Brown, D., and Adams, R. D.: What We Need to Know about Muscle. Neurology 8:65, 1958.

Bielschowsky, A.: Lecture on Motor Anomalies of the Eyes: II. Paralysis of Individual Eye Muscles. Arch. Ophthal. 13:33, 1935; III. Paralysis of Conjugate Ocular Movements. Arch. Ophthal. 13:569, 1935.

Bowden, R. E. M.: A Comparative Study of the Rate of Atrophy of Skeletal Muscle Following Anterior Ramisection and Acute Anterior Poliomyelitis in the Rhesus Monkey. Bull. Hopkins Hosp. 89:153, 1951.

Brock, R. S.: A Study of Miners' Nystagmus. Brit. Med. J. 1:443, 1938.

Brodal, A., and Walberg, F.: Ascending Fibers in Pyramidal Tract of Cat. Arch. Neurol. Psychiat. 68:755, 1952.

Bucy, P. C., ed.: The Precentral Motor Cortex, ed. 2. University of Illinois Press, Urbana, Ill., 1949.

Cogan, D. G.: Accommodation and the Autonomic Nervous System, Arch. Ophthal. 18:739, 1937.

Cogan, D. G.: Neurology of the Ocular Muscles, ed. 2. Charles C Thomas, Springfield, Ill., 1963.

Cox, R. A.: Congenital Head-Nodding and Nystagmus. Arch. Ophthal. 15:1032, 1936.

Critchley, M.: The Parietal Lobes. Williams & Wilkins Co., Baltimore, 1953.

Darley, F. L., Aronson, A. E., and Brown, J. R.: Differential Diagnostic Patterns of Dysarthria. J. Speech Hearing Res. 12:246, 1969.

DeJong, R. N.: Horner's Syndrome. Arch. Neurol. Psychiat. 34:734, 1935.

DeJong, R. N.: The Neurological Examination, ed. 3. Harper & Row, New York, 1967.

DeSchweinitz, G. E.: Concerning Certain Ocular Defects of Pituitary Body Disorders. Trans. Ophthal. Soc. UK 43:12, 1923.

Dix, M. R., Hallpike, C. S., and Hood, J. D.: "Nerve" Deafness: Its Clinical Criteria, Old and New. J. Laryng. Otol. 63:685, 1949.

Duke-Elder, W. S.: Papilledema, in Textbook of Ophthalmology. C. V. Mosby Co., St. Louis, 1941, vol. 3, pp. 2944-2967.

Fischer, J. J.: Otologic Aspects of Vertigo. New Eng. J. Med. 241:142, 1944.

Fischer, J. J.: The Labyrinth. Grune & Stratton, New York, 1956.

Fisher, C. M.: Ocular Bobbing. Arch. Neurol. 11:543, 1964.

Fry, W. F.: Papilledema. Arch. Ophthal. 6:921, 1931.

Fry, W. F.: Pathology of Papilledema. Amer. J. Ophthal. 14:874, 1931.

Harbert, F.: Hearing Loss. Med. Clin. N. Amer. 40:1771, 1956.

Harrington, D. O.: Localizing Value of Incongruity in Defects in the Visual Fields. Arch. Ophthal. 21:453, 1939.

Hines, H. M.: Neuromuscular Denervation, Atrophy and Regeneration. Fed. Proc. 3:231, 1944.

Hughes, B.: The Visual Fields. Charles C Thomas, Springfield, Ill., 1954.

Lambert, E. H.: Neurophysiological Techniques Useful in the Study of Neuromuscular Disorders. Assoc. Res. Nerv. Ment. Dis. Proc. 38:247, 1960.

Lassek, A. M.: The Human Pyramidal Tract. J. Nerv. Ment. Dis. 99:22, 1944.

Lassek, A. M.: The Human Pyramidal Tract. XVIII: An Analysis of its Pathophysiological Status. Brain 73:95, 1950.

Merritt, H. H., and Moore, M.: The Argyll Robertson Pupil. Arch. Neurol. Psychiat. 30:357, 1933.

Nelson, J. R., and Johnston, C. H.: Ocular Bobbing. Arch. Neurol. 22:348, 1970.

Scheie, H. G.: Site of Disturbance in Adie's Syndrome. Arch. Ophthal. 24:225, 1940.

Schwab, R. S., Stafford-Clark, D., and Prichard, J. S.: The Clinical Significance of Fasciculations in Voluntary Muscle. Brit. Med. J. 2:209, 1951.

Smith, J. L., and Cogan, D. G.: Optokinetic Nystagmus in Cerebral Disease. Neurology 10:127, 1960.

Sommer, I., and Yaskin, J. C.: Spontaneous Nystagmus. Arch. Ophthal. 2:57, 1929.

Spiegel, E. A., and Scala, N. P.: Vertical Nystagmus Following Lesions of the Cerebellar Vermis. Arch. Ophthal. 26:661, 1941.

Spiegel, E. A., and Sommer, I.: Neurology of the Eye, Ear, Nose and Throat. Grune & Stratton, New York, 1944.

Spiller, W. G.: Ophthalmoplegia Internuclearis Anterior. Brain 47:345, 1924.

Tower, S.: The Reaction of Muscle to Denervation. Physiol. Rev. 19:1, 1937.

Walsh, F. B.: Clinical Neuro-Ophthalmology, ed. 2. Williams & Wilkins Co., Baltimore, 1957, pp. 276-299.

Walshe, F. M. R., and Robertson, E. G.: Observations upon the Form and Nature of the "Grasping Movements" and "Tonic Innervation" Seen in Certain Cases of Lesions of the Frontal Lobe. Brain 56:40, 1933.

Wartenberg, R.: The Examination of Reflexes. Year Book Publishers, Chicago, 1945.

Wilson, S. A. K.: Problems in Neurology; The Argyll Robertson Pupil. J. Neurol. Psychopath. 2:1, 1921.

Wohlfart, G.: Clinical Considerations on Innervation of Skeletal Muscle. Amer. J. Phys. Med. 38:223, 1959.

CHAPTER 3

The Topical Diagnosis
of Nervous Disease

Neurological diseases become intelligible only if a meaningful relationship can be established between symptoms and signs on the one hand and the precise anatomical localization of the responsible lesion, or lesions, on the other. Localization of the disease process thus becomes the next logical procedure following the examination itself; in fact, if the locus of disease cannot be defined, its very nature may well escape clarification. The process of localization follows logically ordered steps. It should be comprehensible to the student and the generalist as well as to the neurologist; it is this process of localization, i.e., of topical diagnosis, that is of concern herein.

SYMPTOMS OF DEFICIT

Although certain of the symptoms encountered in disease of the nervous system simply reflect loss of function as a direct consequence of a given lesion, e.g., paralysis with interruption of the motor pathway, many others are the expression, not of the diseased or degenerated areas, but of other portions of the brain or spinal cord, the action of which becomes unopposed after the involved areas are thrown out of action. Disease of any portion of the nervous system resulting in loss of cells, or destructive processes of any sort, cannot produce positive symptoms. This was pointed out clearly by Hughlings Jackson, to whom belongs the credit for crystallizing this seemingly obvious principle. Thus, the spasticity and reflex changes that are found in hemiplegia cannot be the expression of an area of destruction of the internal capsule or of any portion of the corticospinal system, since it is obvious that a destroyed area cannot give rise to impulses. In hemiplegia, the impulses conveyed through the corticospinal system are completely interrupted. It follows, therefore, that many of the signs and symptoms of hemiplegia must be the expression of activity of other portions of the neuraxis that act in unopposed fashion after the destroyed area has been shunted out of action; put another way, the clinical manifestations often reflect liberation of lower centers from the control of higher centers. The same holds true for extrapyramidal symptoms associated with paralysis agitans. The positive manifestations of the disease, such as rigidity, tremor, and postural changes, cannot spring directly from a loss of cells in the basal ganglia per se, but must result from the action of other parts of the nervous system that normally act in unison with the diseased areas. Symptoms such as chorea or athetosis, or, in fact, those of disease of any part of the nervous system, must be regarded in the same light. The symptoms resulting from disease of the cerebellum, for example, result probably from unopposed action of the cerebral cortex and brain stem. Positive symptoms cannot, therefore, be produced by negative lesions. The symptoms and signs manifest in any given patient at any point in time therefore represent a combination of symptoms of deficit, such as paralysis or sensory loss, and symptoms of release, such as tremor, rigidity, or hyperreflexia. Understanding of this concept is basic to comprehension of the signs of diseases of the nervous system in the widest sense.

One can do no better than to state the principle involved in the words of Hughlings Jackson. To take hemiplegia as an example, the spasticity in hemiplegia is not the result of the lesion. "There is evidently a duplex symptomatic condition, negative and positive, with loss of power over the muscles, there is tonic action of them. Whilst the primary cerebral lesion can account for the paralytic element—the negative condition—it cannot (nor can the sclerosis in the lateral column) account for the tonic condition of the muscles, the positive element. Negative states of the nervous centers cannot cause positive states of muscles, though they may permit them."

DISTURBANCES OF INTEGRATIVE CEREBRAL FUNCTIONS

Lesions involving the cerebral hemispheres give rise to a number of abnormalities referable, for example, to motility, sensation, and vision, as will be described in detail below. Alterations in higher integrative functions also appear. Changes in mentation, personality, awareness of body organization, etc., have been treated previously (Chapter 2). There remain for consideration here those derangements of symbolic brain function generally referred to as aphasia, agnosia, and apraxia, identification of which is also of major importance in the delineation of hemispheral disease.

Aphasia

Aphasia is loss or impairment of language due to lesions involving specific portions of the brain. It has great localizing value in diagnosis, and if care is

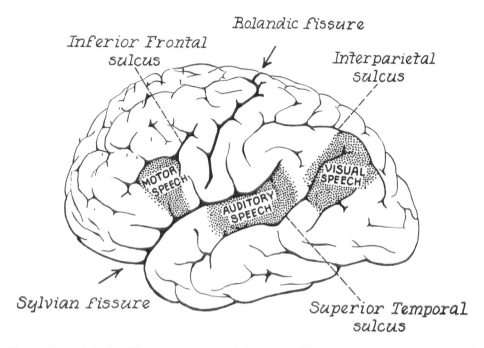

FIGURE 3-1. Aphasia. Diagrammatic view of the principal language areas in the left cerebral hemisphere of a right-handed person. Destruction of the areas indicated is associated with loss of the corresponding language functions.

taken in examination it can be detected fairly readily. Aphasia is a true disorder of symbolic language, and must be distinguished from *dysarthria*, which consists of indistinctness in enunciation of words due to interference with the peripheral speech mechanism (pharynx, larynx, tongue). As already described above, dysarthria occurs with paralysis of the palate; in bulbar paralysis resulting in nasal speech due to palatal immobility; or as indistinctness of speech due to weakness or paralysis of the tongue in hemiplegia, progressive muscular atrophy, or amyotrophic lateral sclerosis; or as indistinct, muffled speech in extra-pyramidal disorders such as paralysis agitans or hepatolenticular degeneration; or in disease of the cerebellum.

Both aphasia and dysarthria must be distinguished from *speech apraxia*, a disorder of speech expression in which the peripheral motor units of speech are intact (unlike dysarthria) but in which these speech mechanisms cannot be used in a coordinated fashion to articulate meaningful phonemes, words, or phrases. Unlike the case in aphasia, symbolic language is preserved, as evidenced by the ability to read and write, and by the absence of a disorder of receptive language. This variety of expressive disorder is generally found with lesions of the inferior frontal convolution and probably accounts for at least some instances of so-called pure expressive aphasia.

Just as a sound vocal apparatus is necessary for normal development and production of speech, so too is a normal receptive mechanism (auditory and visual perception). Kinesthetic and auditory cues (playback) seem to play particularly critical roles in the acquisition of speech; the importance of the latter is especially evident in the speech disorders of the child deaf from birth or an early age.

TESTS FOR APHASIA. Although very severe disorders of language can be readily recognized, accurate diagnosis of more subtle aphasic disturbances requires careful testing at the bedside. A relatively small number of carefully chosen tests, properly applied, will supply much valuable information in this sphere; hasty and haphazardly applied testing, on the other hand, yields only fragmentary and often misleading data of limited value at best. Appropriate bedside testing should include the following:

Spontaneous Speech. If the aphasic patient can be made to speak, he will produce most valuable information. Meticulous attention to spontaneous utterances may prove as informative as the performance of formal language testing; hesitancies in speech, syntactical errors, misuse of words, substitution of words, "word hash," etc., are all apparent in spontaneous speech. It may be difficult or impossible to get an aphasic patient to speak spontaneously. The expressive aphasic is loath to do so because he lacks words, while the auditory-receptive patient is unable to understand requests. Despite this, persistence will yield rich dividends and will enable the examiner to determine whether words are lost or mispronounced, whether word substitutions are made, whether consecutive ideas can be expressed, whether there is complete inability to use words, and what emotional reactions are associated with the effort to express himself.

Auditory Receptive Tests. The understanding of the spoken word can be elicited by various simple tests. It can be done adequately in two ways: (a) By requesting the patient to follow simple commands (put out your tongue, close your eyes, etc.), gradually increasing the complexity of the commands until the patient is dealing with two or more orders (close your eyes and open your mouth; or open your mouth, raise your hand, and close one eye, etc.). (b) By lining up a number of objects that can be produced from any pocket (matches, coin, knife, key, etc.) and by specific commands determining whether the patient understands commands (show me the key, show me the coin, etc.).

Visual Receptive Tests. These can be carried out at the bedside by asking the patient to read from a paper or magazine and to interpret what has been read or by requesting him to follow a few simple written commands. It should be noted whether there is loss of ability to read words or whether there is only mispronunciation of the words read. If the capacity to read is lost, it should be noted whether there is loss of recognition of letters or words, and whether the understanding of words as symbols is impaired or lost.

Writing Test. This is performed easily by asking the patient to write some spontaneous thought and also to write to dictation.

These are only a few of the available tests, but they are sufficient for the bedside examination of the aphasic patient. More extensive and elaborate tests are of relatively limited clinical value but are, of course, essential for investigative purposes.

In the course of detailed testing, the patient with a language disorder may become quite depressed, agitated, and disturbed, often refusing to cooperate further with the examiner. This response has been called a *catastrophic reaction* (Goldstein), and may reflect the patient's increasing awareness of the depth of his disability under the pressure of direct evaluation and observation.

CLASSIFICATION OF APHASIA. All classifications of disorders of language are subject to criticism, in part because it is difficult to achieve a classification that is all inclusive, and in part because any classification tends to create strict and perhaps artificial categories. Four main forms of aphasia are classically recognized, however, and will be utilized here as comprising a prime frame of reference for these disorders. These are: (1) expressive (motor) aphasia, (2) receptive (sensory) aphasia, (3) expressive-receptive (global) aphasia, (4) amnesic (nominal) aphasia. At the outset, it is essential to recognize that these groups refer only to the predominantly affected aspect of speech. *It is extremely rare to find a pure form of language disturbance.* Hence an expressive aphasia is characterized only by predominantly expressive deficits, but auditory-receptive elements are always present. The same holds true of auditory-receptive aphasia. Visual-receptive aphasia, on the other hand, may be found in a pure or almost pure form. At times the predominance of one form of aphasic utterance overshadows only very slightly the other affected form. In all aphasic patients, the extent of the deficit at any given point in time reflects a number of nonspecific factors, such as the patient's mood, interest, familiarity with the test situation, ease of fatigue, length of attention span, and presence and severity of mental confusion. Inconsistency of response is a characteristic feature of many aphasics and reflects to a greater or lesser degree factors such as these.

In general, aphasias develop as a consequence of lesions in the dominant cerebral hemisphere, usually frontotemporal in location and particularly clustering about the insula. In right-handed individuals it is the left hemisphere that is dominant as regards localization of language function. Curiously, the majority of ambidextrous and left-handed individuals also exhibit a dominant left hemisphere, although occasionally right hemispheral dominance is evident. It may not be possible to determine with assurance which hemisphere is dominant on clinical grounds alone; the use of intracarotid Amytal injection may be most informative in this regard.

EXPRESSIVE (MOTOR) APHASIA (BROCA'S APHASIA). This disorder of language is characterized by loss or impairment of power to express oneself, varying in degree from minor difficulty in word finding to virtually complete loss of speech, i.e., mutism. It comprises a defect in language ideation and formulation, in contrast to speech apraxia in which the disorder is one of motility of the speech apparatus, but in which the symbolic functions of language are preserved. The following clinical features may be noted in the patient with expressive aphasia:

Inability to Find Words. Inability to find words with which to express thoughts may consist of occasional loss of a word, evidenced by hesitations in speech, the exact word never being found. In such instances, the lapse may never be filled with the proper word, the patient either passing on after great effort to express himself or bursting into tears or profanity because of his inability to express himself; or he may substitute another word that obviously has no connection with what he is trying to say. It is these cases in which there is occasional loss of words that require recognition. In more advanced cases, words are lost in profusion, the patient being unable to find the name of familiar objects, persons, etc. Retardation in the rate of verbalization may be striking. Dysprosody is often observed, the patient speaking monotonously with little or no inflection or accenting. Simple mispronunciations are frequent, and occasionally defective articulation with frank slurring appears. As a rule, the expressive aphasic will recognize his errors and will attempt to make amends by attempting to find the correct word. In an effort to express his thoughts the patient with expressive aphasia may attempt to form words that sound like those he is seeking (paraphrasia), and for this reason he will make unintelligible words; he may simply substitute one letter for another in a word (hatch for catch, boat for coat, etc.). In addition to substitutions such as these, which are based on phonemic similarities, substitutions may be based on word associations (table for chair, spoon for fork, etc.). The expressive aphasic will often evidence difficulties in the grammatical construction of language and may employ only nouns and verbs, using only an occasional adjective or adverb; this feature, coupled with a tendency to drop out words he cannot find, results in a telegraphic style of communication with remarkable simplification of sentence structure. Word order reversals may also appear, and the patient tends to use words erroneously. In summary, then, the language of the expressive aphasic is characterized by frequent hesitations in speech, with a loss of words resulting in breaks in the continuity of expression and simplification of expression.

The phenomenon of *retained utterances* is particularly noteworthy in the patient with an expressive aphasia. This takes the form of automatic or emotional responses, at times cursing, commonly repeated in stereotyped fashion, appearing unpredictably, and in some severely affected patients comprising the entirety of spoken language. The phrases uttered are often very clearly articulated and at times explosive in quality. They may appear at appropriate times, as during attempts at verbalization, or may emerge inappropriately with no obvious external stimulus. Automatic word series may be evoked, in the form of automatic responses as rote recitations. The automatic phraseology of social intercourse (responses to greetings of good morning, etc.) may also be preserved in aphasia, in both the expressive and receptive varieties.

It is commonly thought that individuals who are multilingual tend to lose the more recently acquired tongue when aphasia develops, reverting thus to their natural speech, though with varying degrees of fluency. This statement probably requires some modification; careful study suggests that in the multilingual patient aphasia develops to an equal degree in all languages equally known, i.e., languages equally known are equally lost. The examiner's own lack of facility in the native language of such patients may, it should be pointed out, contribute to misinterpretation in this regard.

Difficulty in Writing (Dysgraphia). Writing may be regarded as speech recorded on paper; hence the expressive aphasic will show the same disability in his writing as in his speech, the defect ranging from occasional loss of words to complete inability to express himself.

Retention of Understanding through hearing and vision, hence an understanding of both the spoken and written word. This is true only in a broad sense since pure forms of aphasia of any sort are rare. If examined carefully, the patients with expressive aphasia will always demonstrate auditory receptive elements, characterized by difficulty in understanding what is said to them. As indicated above, it is these associated disorders of symbolic language that permit distinction of an expressive aphasia from a speech apraxia.

Expressive aphasia is most commonly the result of a lesion in the posterior part of the third (inferior) frontal convolution (so-called Broca's area) in the dominant, thus usually left, hemisphere.

RECEPTIVE (SENSORY) APHASIA (WERNICKE'S APHASIA). In this type of aphasia, there is predominantly a disturbance or loss in the understanding of speech, the patient finding it difficult or impossible to understand the spoken and often the written word. The outstanding feature of *auditory-receptive aphasia* is disturbance in the understanding of spoken language, the degree depending on the extent of destruction of the area affected. Thus, patients with auditory-receptive aphasia find it difficult or impossible to understand what is said to them. There may be only slight or moderate loss of understanding of words by ear, or there may be virtually total lack of comprehension, the patient failing to respond at all to verbal auditory stimuli. Even in severe cases, however, fragmentary comprehension may be observed at times. In some instances, words seem understood only in a very restricted fashion, with inability to appreciate their full significance, and responses tend to be concrete and simplistic. It should be stressed that the patient with an auditory-receptive aphasia remains capable of hearing sounds and words adequately, the defect being one of comprehension. The patient who fails to respond to all auditory stimuli is either deaf or suffering from auditory agnosia. Involvement of visual language sometimes accompanies receptive aphasia.

Disturbances in expression are commonly encountered in the patient with a receptive aphasia, although of varying severity. One may observe mixing of grammatical constructions, wrong use of words, and substitution of words and even whole phrases in a meaningless sort of jumble. The expressive aphasic, when at a loss for a word, hesitates and fails to produce it; the auditory-receptive-aphasic person, on the other hand, quickly substitutes another and proceeds as if nothing were awry. Unlike the expressive-aphasic person he is unaware of his errors, largely owing to his lack of understanding of auditory impressions, i.e., his lack of the ability to monitor his own (and others') speech; also unlike the expressive aphasic, the amount of verbalization is not reduced, and, in fact, the rate of speech may be greater than normal. Paraphrasing is common, and grammatical confusion and syntactical errors are characteristic. Verbal confusions are frequent; verbal substitutions occur; whole phrases may be inserted in speech in erroneous fashion. As a result, speech in severe cases of auditory-receptive aphasia is likely to be a more or less disjointed and un-intelligible hash; the term *jargon aphasia* is often applied to this state of affairs. Difficulties in *writing* under these circumstances may be as great as those of speech and are of a similar order. Writing, like speech, therefore is inclined to be profuse but confused.

In *visual-receptive aphasia* there is loss of understanding of the printed word and failure to comprehend words as symbols (dyslexia, alexia, word blindness). The capacity to identify letters may be retained, but their synthesis into, and meaning as, words is lost. At times even individual letters fail to be recognized. In defects of a less severe degree, there may be recognition of some or most of the words in a sentence but inability to synthesize the meaning of the sentence. Visual aphasia is often associated with homonymous hemianopsia and with dis-orders of written or spoken language. It may appear as part of the syndrome of *visual object agnosia*, in which not only written symbols but all manner of objects fail to be identified by visual clues alone. A syndrome of pure alexia without agraphia, and without other disturbances of symbolic language, is occasionally en-countered; inability to recognize colors (*color agnosia*) may accompany the read-ing deficit. A curious difference may be noted in the degree of disability as regards reading of letters or words as compared with reading of numbers.

Of considerable interest in the context of visual-receptive aphasia is that condition known as *congenital word blindness,* or *developmental dyslexia.* Al-though of a different order from acquired dyslexia, this inborn and sometimes familial defect may be of great importance in instances of delayed or imperfect acquisition of reading skill in the young. It appears to be a significant though probably uncommon cause of learning disability in the intelligent child without brain damage. A disorder of writing and spatial conceptual defects are sometimes found as associated abnormalities in the dyslexic child.

Auditory-receptive aphasia results from a lesion in the posterior portion of the first (superior) temporal convolution in the dominant hemisphere. The lesion responsible for visual-receptive aphasia tends to be more posteriorly placed, most generally temporo-occipital. Lesions in the splenium of the corpus callosum and in the left visual cortex appear to be critical in the production of the syndrome of pure alexia. The anatomical substrate of developmental dyslexia is unknown.

EXPRESSIVE-RECEPTIVE APHASIA (MIXED OR GLOBAL APHASIA). Cases of this group are characterized by a severe loss of both expressive and receptive elements. The expressive loss is usually so great that only a few sounds or words remain, and the capacity to make even simple sentences is lost. Retained utterances may appear, but the use of automatic phrases is commonly inappro-priate, and true propositional language is lacking. Writing is affected to the same degree as speaking in most cases but may be relatively much better preserved. Understanding of words is greatly limited, the patient failing to understand even single words or simple phrases. The precise location of the lesion responsible for global aphasia cannot be identified with certainty; exten-sive destructive brain lesions are ordinarily noted pathologically.

AMNESIC (NOMINAL) APHASIA (ANOMIA, DYSNOMIA). This type of aphasia consists essentially of difficulty in evoking words as names for objects, conditions or qualities. This difficulty may be so severe that speech is greatly limited. In their motor-speech performance, amnesic aphasics are slow and hesitant and in this respect resemble patients with expressive aphasia, but they show no difficulties in articulation. The amnesic-aphasic patient, unable to find the word for an object, hesitates and substitutes slang or colloquial expressions of many sorts. Rote word series may be employed with ease, but the patient will be unable to evoke isolated and specific items in the series; thus, he may recite the days of the week but be unable to name the current day as a single response. Outstanding in the amnesic defect is the ability of the amnesic-aphasic patient to recognize the word that he himself cannot produce, a characteristic which is not true of the expressive aphasic. Though he recognizes the correct word, and though it is repeated by himself and the examiner often, the amnesic aphasic fails to retain the correct word. The understanding of language is relatively good and reading is fair, although in reading aloud the patient may omit words. Auditory repetition may be impaired, and written language is commonly defective.

The lesion responsible for this variety of language disorder is generally located in the posterior and superior portion of the dominant temporal lobe.

An alternative classification of language disorders is based on linguistics, i.e., on the behavioral attributes of speech and identification of stages of what has been called "phonemic regression." On this basis, several types of aphasia may be identified and may be looked upon as representing various degrees of regression, or reversal, in the normal sequence of language acquisition. Neuroanatomical criteria as such are not utilized. The types of aphasia thus identified are the following:

SYNTACTIC APHASIA. There is a loss of the grammatical function of language, with simplified, concrete, often telegraphic speech. There is little use of connective speech elements, and tense and gender may be improperly used. The use of nominal symbols, i.e., substantive words, is preserved, and communication remains effective. Since the addition of syntax, or grammar, represents the last, or highest, stage in the acquisition of language, this form of aphasia represents the initial level of regression, the first stage of reversal of language function.

SEMANTIC APHASIA. Although grammatical form may be preserved, there is inability to relate the sign to the object, reminiscent of an anomia. Vocabulary restriction may be observed, and circumlocutions are prominent. Less frequently used words tend to be most severely affected. Communication is generally ineffective. This may be looked upon as representing dissolution of the next highest stage of language development, that of the use of substantive (naming) words.

PRAGMATIC APHASIA. This comprises a breakdown in the regulating function of language, the patient being unable to obtain meaning from stimuli and to use such stimuli as a basis for symbol formation. Speech is commonly disordered, with liberal use of paraphrasia and meaningless neologisms; the patient appears unable to perceive his own errors. This seems to correspond to the stage in language development in which the child exhibits aural comprehension but in which oral communication is for the most part fragmentary, ineffective, and contextually meaningless.

JARGON APHASIA. Speech here consists of a profusion of phonemically disorganized combinations of language elements, without understanding on the part of the patient. Reading and writing are seriously impaired. This represents a reversion to the infantile stage of babbling noncommunicative speech (pre-speech).

GLOBAL APHASIA. This is characterized by a lack of linguistic ability, an inability to form verbal symbols for use or in comprehension. Automatic speech and echolalia are sometimes observed. In general, patients so afflicted respond little if at all to environmental stimuli and become totally dependent. Linguistically this represents the first stage of language, i.e., the infantile speechless phase with inability to comprehend or to produce speech.

Aphasias may also be categorized according to the volumetric, quantitative production of speech, i.e., on the basis of fluency. *Fluent* aphasias are characterized by speech that is produced effortlessly, and with good or normal articulation, grammar, rhythm, and prosody, but that is often meaningless and devoid of content. Words are used incorrectly and paraphrasia is commonplace. *Nonfluent* aphasia centers about a very restricted speech output, generally associated with poor articulation and a simplistic telegraphic style. Among the *fluent aphasias* may be recognized: *Wernicke's aphasia*, characterized by inability to understand or repeat verbal symbols, and due to a lesion in the dominant superior temporal region posteriorly (Wernicke's area); *conduction aphasia*, with loss of the ability to repeat words but with preservation of language comprehension, due to a lesion in the suprasylvian parietal white matter (parietal operculum), a lesion effectively disconnecting the receptive from the motor speech areas; *amnestic (anomic) aphasia*, with preservation of powers of both understanding and repetition but difficulty in use of nouns (nominal or substantive words), due at times to a focal lesion in the vicinity of the angular gyrus but also at times encountered as a result of a diffuse encephalopathy; *transcortical aphasia*, due to isolation of the parasylvian speech area from other parts of the cortex, with preservation of powers of repetition but with loss of comprehension. The *nonfluent aphasias* include Broca's *expressive aphasia*, with a lesion in the posterior portion of the inferior frontal convolution (Broca's area), and *global aphasia*, with destruction of both Broca's and Wernicke's areas.

Agnosia

Allied to the problem of aphasia is that of agnosia and apraxia. Agnosia implies the inability to recognize the form or nature of objects. It has been divided into many confusing categories, and attempts have been made to localize each type to a specific part of the cerebral hemisphere, with varying success. The many forms of agnosia described in the medical literature may not in fact themselves represent neatly separable entities, but they are mentioned here to acquaint the student with the variety of forms described.

Tactile agnosia consists of inability to recognize objects by touch and is referred to as *astereognosis*.

Auditory agnosia refers to inability to recognize speech sounds. A special form has been described for musical sounds and is characterized by loss of capacity to recognize tones or melodies (music deafness or *amusia*).

Visual agnosia has been divided into several categories, including agnosia for objects and pictures, or for human faces (the latter being referred to as *prosopagnosia*). In all forms, there is loss of ability to recognize objects or persons by visual cues alone. *Color agnosia* may also be recognized. This is characterized by inability to understand colors as qualities of objects, faulty color concept, and inability to evoke color images, in the absence of color blindness.

Spatial agnosia may be defined as inability to find one's way around familiar places though objects in a room or house are recognized.

Other forms of agnosia are encountered in the context of disorders of the *body image* (see above). A deficit in proprioception and at least mild mental confusion seem common to all these syndromes. The lesions most frequently found in these instances are in the minor (nondominant) parietal lobe. *Anosognosia* consists of ignorance or denial of the existence of disease, usually a lack of perception of a hemiplegia or of other paralyzed parts. There may be imperception of the weakness with a belief by the patient that he can move the paralyzed parts, or a complete denial of the hemiplegia. *Autotopagnosia* (somatotopagnosia, amorphosynthesis) is characterized by loss of ability to identify the body, in whole or in part, or to recognize relationships between the various parts. The patient may, for example, feel an arm next to his body and be unaware that it is his own, or he may be unable to identify sides of the body. *Sensory inattention* may be present for tactile or visual stimuli, or both. In visual inattention, or extinction, the patient can see and recognize objects in any part of the visual field when called upon to do so but will neglect that part of the visual field opposite the side of the lesion when stimuli are presented simultaneously in both halves of the visual field. A similar condition may prevail with touch stimuli.

The *Gerstmann syndrome* is characterized by finger agnosia, agraphia, confusion of right and left, and acalculia. Finger agnosia is expressed by difficulty in recognizing, naming, selecting, and differentiating the fingers of either hand, the patient's own as well as those of others. It involves the middle, ring, and little fingers most severely, the thumb and index less frequently and less severely, and the toes not at all. The confusion of right and left is characterized by inability to recognize sides of the body, both the patient's as well as others. The acalculia is seen as a difficulty, often profound, in performing simple arithmetical problems. The syndrome is most commonly due to a lesion involving the left angular gyrus in a right-handed person, in the region between the parietal and occipital cortex.

Although not strictly speaking an agnosia, the syndrome of the *phantom limb* (or phantom nose, breast, penis) may be looked upon as an unawareness or lack of recognition of a loss of part of the body and, in a certain light, as an unconscious attempt to preserve the integrity of the body image. Patients so afflicted experience positive phenomena, generally tactile or proprioceptive in quality, at the site of the missing part. The limb is felt as present, though often painful and in stressed or distorted postures. With the passage of time shrinkage and ultimately disappearance of the phantom occur. No lesions of the central nervous system are demonstrable under these circumstances; abnormal activity on the part of peripheral nerve trunks sectioned during amputation appears to be responsible for the appearance of the phantom, but the precise events leading to conscious awareness of a lost part are not known.

Apraxia

This form of disorder refers to inability to perform purposeful movements or to execute the proper use of objects. Several forms are described:

Limb kinetic, characterized by absence of paralysis, slowness, awkwardness, and generally inability to carry out a movement.

Ideokinetic, evidenced by difficulty in determining what the movement shall be.

Ideational, demonstrated by inability to recognize the specific movements necessary for the completion of an act. Patients so afflicted are unable altogether to strike a match and light a cigarette, or they may strike the match on the wrong side of the box, or strike with the cigarette instead of the match.

Constructional, in which difficulty in building with blocks, in drawing, and sometimes in writing is encountered. The patient may be aware of the faulty nature of his efforts. Design copying may be similarly affected. At times, only half the constructions, or drawings, are defective, almost always the left half, indicating a primary visuospatial problem with neglect of the left side of extracorporeal space.

Dressing apraxia, typified by failure of the patient to clothe himself correctly. As most commonly found, it is the left side that remains partially or totally unclad, as an expression of *neglect* of the left side of the body. Both dressing and constructional apraxia appear most commonly with lesions of the right, or nondominant, parietal lobe.

Speech apraxia has already been alluded to in the discussion of expressive aphasia. It is sometimes considered part of a more widespread practic disorder called *facial apraxia*. Lesions of the inferior and posterior portion of the dominant frontal lobe are considered the cause of this affection.

Gait apraxia, generally thought to be a reflection of disease of the frontal lobes, comprises an inability to utilize the limbs in an effective and coordinated fashion when erect in terms of walking; when the patient is tested in a recumbent position, however, the legs appear normal.

Clinical Significance of Aphasia, Agnosia, and Apraxia

Defects in speech of the aphasic type have an important clinical significance and indicate lesions in specific portions of the brain. Care must be taken, however, to recognize the fact that, as Hughlings Jackson has said, "To locate the damage which destroys speech and to locate speech are two different things." Hence the localization of lesions causing aphasia fails to state how the speech process is elaborated. Categorically stated, expressive aphasia indicates a lesion in the left inferior frontal gyrus in its posterior portion and possibly also implicates the adjacent island of Reil (insula). Auditory-receptive aphasia indicates a lesion in the posterior portion of the left superior temporal gyrus. Visual-receptive aphasia indicates a lesion in the region of the lingual gyrus or, when found in pure form, in the splenium of the corpus callosum and the occipital cortex. In the expressive-receptive group, there is involvement of both frontal and temporal areas. The localization in the amnesic group is not clear, but a posterior and superior temporal locus is probable.

The localizing significance of the practic and gnostic disorders is perhaps less clear cut. In general, the lesions responsible for the agnosias are parietal or temporo-occipital. Apraxias of the speech, facial, and gait varieties accompany frontal lesions, whereas constructional and dressing apraxias appear as a result of parietal lesions. Idiokinetic and ideational forms seem dependent on lesions of the corpus callosum for their appearance. The significance of isolation, or separation, of one part of the cerebrum from the remainder in the pathogenesis of disorders of this type has recently been re-emphasized by Geschwind, who defines three major groups of so-called *disconnection syndromes*:

1. *Commissural syndrome*. Following destruction of all, or nearly all, of the corpus callosum surgically or as a consequence of anterior cerebral artery occlusion, a variety of clinical defects emerge, which include inability to match a stimulus object held in one hand with the other, or seen on one visual field with the other; inability to carry out verbal commands with the left hand, though able to do so with the right; inability to write with the left hand, although writing with the right hand is preserved; inability to name objects held in the left hand; inability to read in the left visual field; constructional apraxia; abnormalities of dichotic listening. If the lesion is restricted to the splenium of the corpus callosum alone, inability to read or name objects in the left visual field may be observed as an isolated deficit.

2. *Conduction aphasia*. This syndrome appears as a result of a lesion interrupting intra-hemispheral associational systems, specifically the internal arcuate fasciculus in the parietal operculum, that fiber system which connects Wernicke's area in the superior temporal gyrus and Broca's area in the frontal lobe; both Wernicke's and Broca's areas themselves are spared. The aphasia is of the fluent variety (see above), with paraphrasia, and is associated with dysgraphia and severe impairment of the ability to repeat verbally-presented phrases. Despite the disorder of repetition, the understanding of spoken and written speech is normal, or nearly so. A right hemisensory defect is often found. The aphasic disorder is felt to reflect the disconnection of Wernicke's from Broca's area. Apraxia may also be observed in patients so affected, with difficulty in executing movements with either side in response to verbal commands.

3. *Disorders resulting from commissural lesions combined with others*, including:

a. Alexia without agraphia. Generally associated with a right homonymous hemianopsia and defective color naming, this syndrome appears as a result of a combination of lesions in the left visual cortex and in the splenium of the corpus callosum. So-called mind blindness, characterized by inability to identify or select objects visually, may occur with lesions similarly placed.

b. Apraxia of the left side with Broca's aphasia. A right hemiparesis is usually present as well. This results from a lesion involving either the arcuate fibers as they enter the premotor region in the dominant hemisphere, or the origin of the callosal fibers. A similar clinical deficit may appear with a single large subcortical infarction.

c. Pure word deafness. This consists of difficulty in comprehension of spoken language, with normal hearing, normal identification of nonverbal sounds, and virtually normal speech, reading, and writing. It has been described under two circumstances: either as a result of bilateral lesions affecting the first temporal gyrus, or of a subcortical left temporal lobe lesion sparing Wernicke's area but implicating the left auditory radiation and the callosal fibers from the right auditory region, thus essentially disconnecting Wernicke's area from auditory stimulation.

d. Isolation of the speech area, or transcortical aphasia. Here comprehension and production of speech are impaired, but powers of repetition are preserved. This appears due to a lesion in which Wernicke's and Broca's areas, and the interconnecting arcuate fasciculus, are preserved, in the face of extensive destruction of both gray and white matter elsewhere in the cerebrum.

LESIONS INVOLVING THE VISUAL SYSTEM

The visual fibers are distributed in orderly arrangement throughout their course. Impulses are brought to the retina from the visual field, stimuli from the temporal field arriving at the nasal side of the retina, those from the nasal field, the temporal side. Stimuli from the upper portion of the visual field fall on the lower part of the retina; those from the lower portions, on the upper part of the retina. Fibers from the temporal side of the retina (nasal field) pass through the nerve and optic chiasm uncrossed, while those from the nasal side (temporal field) cross through the chiasm. In the chiasm the ratio of crossed to uncrossed fibers is 3:2. Fibers from the upper part of the retina lie in the upper part of the optic nerve and chiasm; those from the lower retina, in the lower part of the optic nerve and chiasm. The visual fibers then continue to the primary optic centers, the external geniculate bodies. Thence they continue as the optic radiation, hooking around the inferior horn of the lateral ventricle as the geniculocalcarine radiation. Here the fibers are closely packed together, passing through the temporal and occipital lobes, fanning out more and more as they proceed to their final end stations in the calcarine cortex of the occipital lobe, which has an upper and lower lip. Fibers from the upper half of the retina (lower half of visual field) are distributed to the upper calcarine lip; those from the lower half of the retina (upper half of the visual field), to the lower calcarine lip.

The papillomacular bundle, which subserves central vision, runs from the macular region to the external geniculate body and from there to the cortex. It lies roughly in the center of the optic nerve and chiasm and is distributed to the more superior portions of the geniculate. The macula is projected onto the tip of the occipital lobe; hence a lesion here will cause loss of central vision. Because of the frequent escape of central vision with resultant preservation of visual acuity in complete hemianopsias, it has been suggested that there is bilateral representation of the macula in the striate area, and it is believed by some that macular fibers cross in the splenium of the corpus callosum. Others assume a diffuse representa-

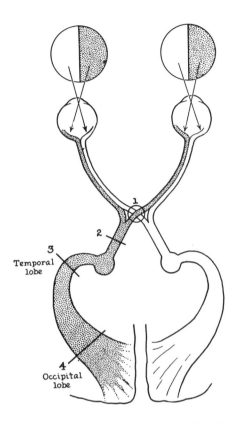

FIGURE 3-2. Visual fields indicating the origin and destination of the visual pathways showing the crossed and uncrossed fibers. Lesions at 1 produce bitemporal hemianopsia. Lesions at 2, 3, and 4 produce homonymous hemianopsia. Lesions at 2 and 3 are more apt to produce field cuts with involvement of the fixation points.

tion of the macula in the striate area. Such sparing of central vision in most hemianopsias, however, may simply reflect a different pattern of blood supply (middle vs. posterior cerebral arteries) in the tip of the occipital lobe (macular area) as compared with the remainder of the calcarine cortex.

The form of the visual field itself is flattened above and restricted medially by the bony ridges of the orbit and the bridge of the nose. Hence it is not a complete circle. Its form is affected also by the width of the palpebral fissure, the size of the pupil, and the visual acuity.

The visual fields are composed of binocular and monocular portions because of the position of the eyes in the head and the overlapping of the fields of vision. The binocular portions extend out to 60 degrees of the visual field. In each visual field on the temporal side (60 to 90 degrees) is a portion known as the temporal crescent, concerned with monocular vision.

Visual Field Syndromes

These have already been discussed in detail (see above), and will be reviewed here only in outline form:

SCOTOMAS. Scotomas develop as a result of lesions of the retina, or of the optic nerve between the eye and the chiasm. They may be central, paracentral or cecocentral. The most common is the central scotoma associated with retrobulbar neuritis; here, visual acuity is decreased. Multiple sclerosis is a common cause, but any condition affecting the optic nerve, such as a suprasellar meningioma compressing the optic nerve anterior to the chiasm, will produce a scotoma.

ALTITUDINAL ANOPSIA. This rare defect is characterized by loss of vision in the upper or lower halves of the visual fields and is due to a lesion anterior to the optic chiasm pressing on the upper or under surfaces of the optic nerves.

BINASAL HEMIANOPSIA. A loss of both nasal fields is due to involvement of the uncrossed fibers coming from the temporal part of the retinae. It results only from bilateral lesions, almost always sclerosed, tortuous, and dilated (ectatic) internal carotid arteries. It has been described with pituitary tumor.

BITEMPORAL HEMIANOPSIA. This common field defect results from compression or destruction of the decussating fibers in the center of the optic chiasm derived from the nasal sides of the retinae. The visual loss usually extends cleanly through the fixation point, but often with sparing of central vision. It is caused by many lesions involving the optic chiasm, chief among which are intrasellar tumors (pituitary adenomas), and suprasellar lesions such as meningiomas, hypophyseal stalk tumors, and aneurysms. A localized form of thickening of the leptomeninges, so-called chiasmatic arachnoiditis, is implicated in some cases. It may occasionally be caused by compression of the chiasm from above due to a dilated third ventricle or to a third ventricle tumor.

HOMONYMOUS HEMIANOPSIA. This is the most common field defect encountered. It consists of a loss of vision in the temporal field of one eye and the nasal field of the other and is found with lesions of all sorts that affect the optic tract and radiation. Homonymous hemianopsia in itself has no localizing value except to indicate involvement of the opposite tract or radiation, decision as to temporal, occipital, or parasellar (tract) involvement depending upon the presence of other symptoms.

RETINAL FIELD DEFECTS. For purposes of comparison, brief mention may here be made of at least some of the visual defects encountered with disease of the *retina* itself rather than of the conducting apparatus. Conditions as divergent as neuronal storage disease (Tay-Sachs) or chorioretinitis may involve the macula, resulting in a *central scotoma* with impairment of visual acuity. Focal destructive lesions elsewhere in the retina, as seen for example in instances of retinal hemorrhage or separation, produce delimited *sector* field cuts generally corresponding in an anatomical sense to the diseased portion of the retina. Visual acuity is preserved if the macular area is spared. *Peripheral constriction* of the fields may be found in disorders that destroy retinal ganglion cells in diffuse fashion, as in methyl alcohol intoxication. A loss of night vision, or *night blindness*, is the first sign of *retinitis pigmentosa*, characterized by degeneration of the peripheral rod-bearing portions of the retina; as the disease progresses, increasing limitation of the fields ensues, and ultimately optic atrophy and blindness result. Night blindness is also the characteristic visual abnormality of *vitamin A deficiency*, and here too is referable to dysfunction of the rods; lack of vitamin A results in a lack of retinene, and thus rhodopsin (visual purple), the photosensitive agent of the rods.

LESIONS OF THE UPPER MOTOR NEURON

The term upper motor neuron indicates any central neuron conveying impulses to the anterior horn cell. Lesions may affect this neuron anywhere from the cerebral cortex to the anterior horn cell of the spinal cord. The most important pathway concerned is the corticospinal (pyramidal tract), which takes its origin in the cells of the cortex, passes through the internal capsule, the cerebral peduncle, and pons, decussates low in the medulla, and passes down the cord in the lateral columns, synapsing eventually with anterior horn cells.

Not all of the fibers of the corticospinal or pyramidal tract are derived from the Betz cells of the precentral gyrus; it is probable that the parietal lobe makes important contributions to the pyramidal tract, but the precise portions contributed by this or other portions of the cortex are not definitely defined. Corticospinal

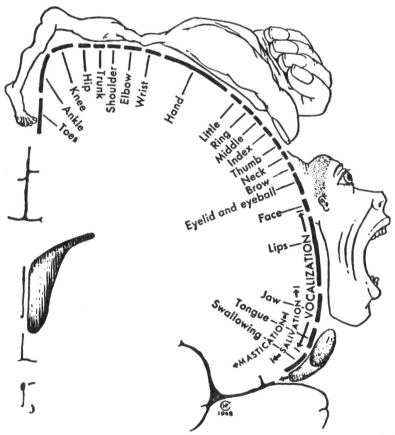

FIGURE 3-3. Motor homunculus, showing the representation of the various parts of the body in the motor cortex. The face, hand, and foot areas are most widely represented. (From Penfield, W., and Rasmussen, T.: The Cerebral Cortex of Man: A Clinical Study of Localization of Function, 1950. By permission of The Macmillan Co.)

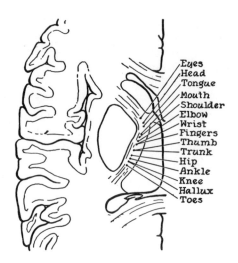

FIGURE 3-4. Internal capsule, showing in diagram form the situation of
the fibers to the various portions of
the limbs and trunk of the opposite
side of the body.

fibers originating in the precentral gyrus and the parietal lobe comprise the best known group of fibers in the pyramids, accounting for 50 per cent of the axons therein. Whether the remaining 50 per cent of fibers are of cortical or subcortical origin is uncertain. Since about half the fibers in the pyramid remain intact after hemispherectomy, it is presumed that subcortical levels contribute a significant portion thereto. In this connection, it is interesting to note that there are 25,000 to 30,000 Betz cells in the motor cortex and about 1 million axons in the pyramid. Only about 10 to 15 per cent, incidentally, achieve direct synaptic connection with anterior horn cells; the majority end in relation to cells in the intermediate zone. A variety of other upper motor neuron impulses also play upon the anterior horn cell, including rubrospinal, tectospinal, reticulospinal, and olivospinal pathways.

Interruption of the corticospinal pathway for any reason results in paralysis of the opposite side of the body, known as *hemiplegia*. The face may or may not participate, depending on the segmental level of the lesion responsible. When both corticospinal pathways are interrupted in the brain, *diplegia* results, as in the cerebral diplegia of children. If a single limb or a focal portion of the body (face) is affected, the result is *monoplegia*. At lower levels *paraplegia* develops, involving usually the legs; when both arms and legs are affected, the term *quadriplegia* is utilized.

As indicated, the name "paraplegia" is customarily used to refer to paralysis of the legs, but it could be used for paralysis of the arms as well (brachial paraplegia). It is associated as a rule with bilateral pyramidal tract disease in the spinal cord, but it may result from focal bilateral disease of the motor cortex or the internal capsules or of the corticospinal pathway in the brain stem. In the majority of cases, paraplegia is in extension with weakness of the legs, spasticity, extensor plantar responses, etc. It most frequently results from lesions that gradually compress or destroy the cord.

When it develops acutely, as in cases of spinal cord injury or in acute transection from other causes, the paraplegia is flaccid, a manifestation of the syndrome of *spinal shock*; spasticity ordinarily appears with the passage of time. Spastic paraplegia may be recognizable when the patient walks, the gait characteristically being shuffling as a result of the increased extensor tonus. On recumbency, spasticity usually persists but in some cases disappears, to be elicited again in walking.

In some instances a *paraplegia in flexion* develops. In such cases the legs develop involuntary flexor spasms, elicited by touching the foot, stroking the skin, lifting the bedclothes, etc. The flexor spasms are followed by involuntary extension after a varying time. The result is alternating flexion and extension occurring at irregular intervals. These eventually give way to complete flexion paraplegia. The legs are paralyzed in the final stages of the disorder; the patellar reflexes cannot as a rule be elicited because of the marked flexor rigidity, and the withdrawal reflexes are greatly exaggerated. This state of affairs has been reported in spinal cord tumor, multiple sclerosis, and spinal cord syphilis, and in fact is likely to be seen in any longstanding paraplegia associated with complete or incomplete interruption of the spinal cord pathways. It is presumably the result of

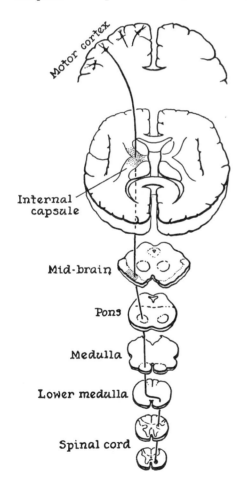

FIGURE 3-5. Corticospinal tract indicating its origin and destination around the anterior horn cells.

dysfunction of an extrapyramidal path in the spinal cord, since it does not follow pure pyramidal tract interruption.

If only portions of the corticospinal pathway are diseased or injured, *monoplegia* may result. This is manifested by a focal loss of power in the opposite side of the body, thus resulting in facial weakness or weakness of a hand (manual monoplegia), or of an arm (brachial monoplegia), or of face, tongue, and arm (facio-lingual-brachial monoplegia). The number of possible combinations is great, depending upon the area affected. Monoplegias result almost always from disease of the motor cortex but in rare instances may result from involvement of the corticospinal pathway itself.

Signs of Upper Motor Neuron Lesion

This is characterized by the following group of symptoms:

PARALYSIS. In a typical instance this involves the opposite face, arm, and leg, the precise distribution of course reflecting the site of the lesion. In some cases, face, palate, tongue, arm, and leg may be involved. The chest and abdominal muscles on the affected side are implicated; in fresh hemiplegias it is possible to detect weakness of the abdominal muscles, which are hypotonic and fail to contract as well as those of the healthy side. The paralysis is usually *spastic*, the spasticity standing in contrast to the flaccid paralysis of lower motor neuron disease. It is characterized by an increase of muscle tone of a "clasp-knife" variety, passive movement of a muscle resulting first in an increase of the muscle tone, followed, as one continues, by a sudden release. In some cases only uniform resistance to passive movement is present, without frank spasticity. With the usual spastic hemiparesis, the affected limbs assume a characteristic attitude, with varying degrees of flexion of the elbow, wrist, and fingers, pronation of the forearm, and adduction of the shoulder, along with an extended posture of the leg. Typically, the distal muscles are involved by weakness to a greater extent than the proximal; thus, in the arms, fingers and hand movements are severely affected, movements of the forearm, upper arm, and shoulder much less so. With discrete lesions in the motor cortex, however, very focal deficits may appear, reflecting the precise somatotopic representation evident there. Somewhat less discrete topographical representation is found in the internal capsule, and small lesions here may also result in quite restricted deficits.

Paralysis due to interruption of the corticospinal tract is not always spastic. As has been pointed out, it may be completely flaccid with an acutely evolving lesion. Under such circumstances, the flaccidity may be transient or permanent. The cause of flaccidity with upper motor neuron lesions is not definitely known, and its occurrence with lesions of the cerebral hemispheres constitutes a thorny problem. In the experimental animal, particularly primates, ablation restricted to the motor strip (Area 4) results in flaccid hemiplegia, with little change in reflex activity (though with an extensor plantar sign, at least in the chimpanzee). If premotor (4s) cortex is included, moderate spasticity is observed, along with increase in the tendon reflexes. If the lesion includes still more anteriorly placed cortex (Area 6), marked spasticity with extreme hyper-reflexia results. (In this connection, established projections of Areas 4, 4s, and 6 to a wide variety of extra-pyramidal structures such as caudate, putamen, substantia nigra, subthalamic nucleus, red nucleus, reticular formation, and pontine nuclei are worthy of note.) Unfortunately, comparable data are not available for man, since pure motor or premotor cortical lesions are very rare. One cannot assert with assurance, as is possible in the experimental animal, that lesions confined to the motor cortex result in flaccid hemiplegia. Spastic hemiplegia is more commonly encountered in human material, most frequently associated with (deep) lesions involving the capsule. Such evidence as is available would suggest that spasticity resulting from lesions of the corticospinal system is actually due to unopposed (released) activity of some other, extrapyramidal, part of the brain and, thus, a manifestation of extrapyramidal rather than pyramidal action. Walshe may be quoted in this regard: "From clinical and experimental sources come several indications, as yet imperfectly understood, that a pure cortical lesion of the pyramidal system often does not produce spasticity as an accompaniment of the loss of power. They suggest the possibility that in the cerebral lesion underlying, for example, a typical spastic residual hemiplegia, analysis may ultimately reveal a second component. That is, in addition to a negative lesion of the corticospinal path, interruption of another descending path may be concerned in the production of spasticity. Such a path need not necessarily be cerebrospinal."

BULBAR AFFECTION IN HEMIPLEGIA. Facial paralysis appears in cortico-spinal lesions. It involves only the lower part of the face and is shown by slow-ness and weakness in retraction of the mouth and flattening of the normal angulation of the mouth and of the nasolabial fold on the affected side (central facial weakness). The palate may be paralyzed on one side, manifested by droop-ing of the affected side, with pulling of the palate to the healthy side on phonation. The tongue may also be involved and is pushed over to the paralyzed side on protrusion. The mechanism of production of cranial nerve palsies in hemiplegia is understandable if one considers the anatomy involved. The motor nuclei of the brain stem receive innervation from the motor cortex through the corticobulbar tract, which conveys impulses to the motor cranial nerve nuclei from above (supranuclear innervation). The tract forms part of the corticospinal sys-tem but as a separate bundle. Fibers to the face are conveyed through this tract, the forehead and eyelids being innervated bilaterally, while the lower portion of the face receives only unilateral innervation. For this reason only the lower portion of the face is paralyzed as a result of a unilateral corticospinal lesion. Most other bulbar motor functions, such as phonation and chewing, receive bilateral innerva-tion and are, therefore, not affected in corticospinal disease. Movements of the palate and tongue, however, may be affected with unilateral lesions.

INCREASE OF TENDON REFLEXES. The tendon reflexes of the paralyzed side (biceps, triceps, patellar, Achilles reflexes) are overactive in corticospinal lesions, presumably as the result of release of the anterior horn cells from the inhibitory effects of the corticospinal pathway. Thus, like the spasticity, over-active reflexes are an expression of extrapyramidal influences. Generally speak-ing, the reflexes are increased in proportion to the spasticity. However, muscles may be so spastic as to produce no response and, contrariwise, flaccidity of corti-

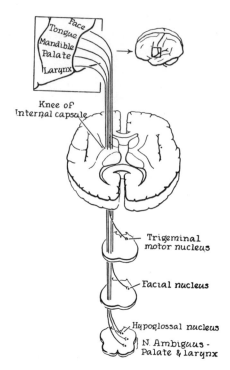

FIGURE 3-6. Corticospinal tract, showing the projection of the corticobulbar pathways on the motor nuclei of the brain stem.

cospinal disease may be associated with overactive reflexes. *Clonus* of the muscles is frequently found along with the increased muscle tone. Most common is ankle clonus, but patellar, wrist, and even pectoral clonus may be encountered. Clonus consists of a repetitive movement of the muscles, a rhythmic reappearance of contraction after stimulation. Ankle clonus is elicited by quick, vigorous dorsiflexion of the foot, with the knee held in flexion. The sought-for result in cases of corticospinal disease is a repeated or clonic movement of the foot maintained so long as the foot is held firmly in dorsiflexion. Ordinarily, the clonus stops when the foot is released, but it may continue spontaneously, ceasing only with vigorous plantar flexion. Spontaneous clonus at the ankle may develop in cases of advanced spasticity. Patellar clonus is elicited by vigorous downward movement of the patella with the leg in full extension; wrist clonus, by vigorous extension of the wrist.

LOSS OF CUTANEOUS REFLEXES. A frequent feature of corticospinal disease is the loss of the cutaneous reflexes, notably the abdominal and cremasteric, on the side of the paralysis. They are lost bilaterally in paraplegia. Impairment of these superficial reflexes is not invariable. The corneal reflex may be decreased or absent in acute hemiplegia, returning with recovery.

The mechanism of loss of the superficial reflexes in hemiplegia is not clearly understood. The basic reflex arc concerned at least in loss of the abdominal reflex would appear to be spinal. Since there is no evidence of abnormality at the spinal or peripheral level in the typical hemiplegic, it must be assumed that the decrease in response is due to deficiency in excitatory volleys derived from higher centers.

ABNORMAL OR PATHOLOGICAL REFLEXES. The most important and the most significant of the abnormal reflexes with corticospinal disease is the extensor plantar response of Babinski (Babinski's sign). This is pathognomonic of corticospinal disease. Although Babinski's sign never occurs without corticospinal disease, at least after infancy, the converse is not necessarily true, and corticospinal disease may be found without a Babinski sign. This and other pathological responses have been described in detail (Chapter 2).

In many cases, all signs listed are easily elicited. In other instances, various combinations may be encountered. Only slight weakness of one side may be present (hemiparesis). There may be only very slight weakness associated with increased reflexes with or without abnormal reflexes; or there may be a Babinski sign without other evidence of corticospinal disease; or weakness may be present with only slightly increased reflexes. These slight or partial manifestations of corticospinal disease are very important to recognize. It is well to bear in mind that a positive Babinski sign always means corticospinal disease, even as an isolated observation.

It is often necessary to differentiate a hemiplegia of structural or organic origin from one of psychogenic origin. Of basic importance is the personality structure, which is found to be consistent with a psychogenic reaction. The history is often helpful, particularly in regard to onset of the weakness and the circumstances surrounding it. Most important, however, are the discrepancies revealed on examination. There may be good finger dexterity despite hand weakness; balancing on the weak leg may be quite normal; walking fails to reveal the typical hemiplegic gait; the weak arm has no difficulty in performing rapid alternating and patting tests; the reflexes are not increased; and there are no pathological reflexes.

LESIONS OF THE LOWER MOTOR NEURON

Lesions of the lower motor neuron, i.e., of the motor side of the reflex arc, may involve (1) the anterior horn cells, (2) the anterior roots, (3) the peripheral nerve, or, in other words, the peripheral neuron anywhere from its cell of origin (anterior horn cell) outward. Common symptoms of deficit arise whether the interruption be at the anterior horn cell, anterior root, or motor peripheral nerve. It may be possible to differentiate the various levels of involvement, but the fact remains that in lesions of the anterior horn cell and the motor system "downstream" from it the majority of the clinical features are identical. All lesions on the motor side of the reflex arc produce paralysis, atrophy of the affected muscle or muscles in varying degree, loss or decrease of reflexes, and changes in the electromyogram.

Anterior Horn Cell Syndrome

The features of anterior horn cell disease hold true for involvement of the anterior horn cells of the spinal cord or brain stem (motor cranial nerve nuclei), regardless of the specific variety of disease concerned (poliomyelitis, amyotrophic lateral sclerosis, syringomyelia, progressive muscular atrophy, etc.) The syndrome is characterized by: (1) *Paralysis*. This is always flaccid and hypotonic, segmental in character, and either partial or complete for a particular muscle or group of muscles, depending on the number of anterior horn cells destroyed. (2) *Atrophy*. This is always present and depends in degree on the number of cells destroyed. It may follow soon after paralysis occurs or it may be delayed. (3) *Fasciculations*. These occur as part of the anterior horn cell syndrome and when present establish the diagnosis of anterior horn cell disease. They are not always seen, however, because of total atrophy of the muscle or obscuration by overlying fat. (4) *Loss of reflexes*. This occurs as the result of interruption of the reflex arc. (5) *Fibrillation potentials* and other evidence of denervation with electromyography. (6) *Absence of sensory disturbances*. Since the anterior horn cells are purely motor in function, sensory disturbances are completely lacking.

PATHOGENESIS. The pathogenesis of the various features of disease of the anterior horn cells is a matter of great practical interest. The *paralysis* that invariably accompanies the disease is the direct result of loss of innervation of the muscles due to interruption of the motor fibers at their cell of origin. It is obvious that if all the cells innervating a muscle or muscles are destroyed the paralysis will be complete; if the anterior horn cell destruction is incomplete the degree of paralysis will depend on the number of cells destroyed and therefore the number of fibers interrupted. Study of the innervation ratio, that is, the proportion of nerve to muscle fibers in lower animals, indicates that in extensor longus digitorum, for example, the ratio is 1:165 and in soleus 1:120. This means that when one anterior horn cell to soleus is stimulated an average of 120 muscle fibers is thrown into action; consequently, the loss of even a single anterior horn cell by disease will result in appreciable loss of power in the affected muscle. A single anterior horn cell can also be shown capable, with repetitive discharge, of developing an average of 30 gm. of tension in the gastrocnemius, another sign of the significance of a single cell in this regard.

An important feature of anterior horn cell paralysis is its *segmental character*. The spinal cord is a chain of segments operating through separate reflex arcs interacting with one another. Each segment of the spinal cord bears a specific relationship to a definite sensory and motor segment of the body. From the motor side, specific muscles are innervated through specific segments of the spinal cord. Muscles may be innervated through a single cord segment or, as is more usual, through two or three segments. Thus, through segments C5 and C6 in the cervical cord are innervated biceps, deltoid, part of the pectoralis major, teres major and minor, serratus magnus, supraspinatus, infraspinatus, rhomboids, subscapularis, and the flexor muscles of the hand. A lesion involving these segments, therefore, will result in complete or partial paralysis of the affected muscles, or, in other words, a segmental type of paralysis. The same group of muscles may be affected by simultaneous involvement of their respective peripheral nerves, but the resulting features differ from those of anterior horn cell disease. It does not follow, of course, that in disease of a specific segment or segments all the muscles innervated through these segments will be paralyzed. Some may be affected and others not. Since in addition the atrophy associated with anterior horn cell disease may be so extensive and diffuse that its segmental character cannot be identified, the segmental nature of anterior horn cell involvement may be of more theoretical than practical significance.

The *atrophy* resulting from anterior horn cell disease is still unexplained in many details. Intact innervation is essential for the maintenance of normal muscle bulk, and anatomical continuity of the nerve is important in preventing atrophy. According to some, atrophy results from the overactivity of the muscles as a result of the constant fasciculations or fibrillations following denervation; however, repeated doses of quinidine and atropine abolish or inhibit fibrillary activity but have no effect on atrophy, and conversely drugs that increase fibrillary activity (neostigmine, acetylcholine, Mecholyl) do not affect the atrophy. Electrical stimulation is effective in delaying atrophy, and it would appear that the maintenance of muscle tension and activity is of great importance in preventing muscle atrophy. The time of development of atrophy after anterior horn cell disease varies considerably, although the factors responsible for differences in the rate are not known (Table 3-1). In some instances it develops rapidly as in poliomyelitis; in others more slowly, as in progressive muscular atrophy and amyotrophic lateral sclerosis. From a clinical standpoint it seems that the extent of atrophy parallels the destruction of anterior horn cells.

Anterior Root Syndrome

This is indistinguishable from that of the anterior horns.

Motor Peripheral Nerve Syndrome

Some peripheral nerves are exclusively or almost exclusively motor in function (radial, long thoracic nerve, etc.). Disease of such nerves may give rise to syndromes similar to those of anterior horn cell disease. The main clinical characteristics are: (1) paralysis, which, as is the case in all peripheral nerve syndromes, is always flaccid; (2) atrophy of the muscle or muscles supplied by the affected nerve; (3) loss of reflexes; (4) electromyographic evidence of denervation; (5) absence of pain; (6) absence of sensory disturbances. They differ, however, in the following respects; (a) The atrophy is, as a rule, less extensive and severe, and develops less rapidly. In a completely interrupted nerve, however, it may be as intense as in anterior horn cell disease. (b) There are usually no fasciculations. In those instances in which fasciculations are found in peripheral nerve disease, the assumption is often made that there is coexistent anterior horn cell disease. Apart from these differences the findings are similar.

Mixed Peripheral Nerve Syndrome

Since most nerves contain both motor and sensory fibers, syndromes involving the peripheral nerves are most commonly of a mixed type. Not all the features of a mixed peripheral nerve syndrome are found in the same degree in all instances of involvement of the nerve, variability depending on such factors as the nature of the causative agent and the degree of damage of the nerve. The symptoms

Table 3-1.   Rate of Atrophy of Skeletal Muscle

(*Summary of Work Compiled from Literature*)

1. DENERVATION
   (1) *Rabbits*
      Began 3-7 days.
      Established and progressed, 14-63 days (2-9 weeks).
   (2) *Rats*
      Evident 3-10 days.
      Established and progressed, 14 days on.
   (3) *Monkeys*
      Evident 7 days.
      Established and progressed, 84 days (12 weeks).

2. TENOTOMY
   (1) *Rabbits*
      Evident 2 weeks.
   (2) *Rats*
      Evident 7-10 days.
      Established and progressed, 17 days.

3. DISUSE
   Monkeys
   Evident 1 week.
   Established and progressed, 10 weeks.

4. ANTERIOR RAMISECTION
   Monkeys
   Evident 10 days.

consist of: (1) *Pain:* When present this immediately differentiates the syndrome from pure anterior horn cell involvement, since the latter is purely motor in function. It may be quite intense, as in alcoholic (nutritional) or diabetic neuropathy, or with peripheral nerve tumors, but many neuropathies are relatively pain free. The pain is felt along the distribution of the peripheral nerve affected; it is constant and usually severe and may be relieved by heat. (2) *Tenderness of the nerves, muscles,* and *tendons:* Tenderness of the nerves is almost always present but it varies in degree; in some cases it is severe, in others only moderate or mild. Usually muscle tenderness is present in the region of the muscles supplied by the affected nerve, but it may be absent or very mild in degree. While nerve and muscle tenderness is always found in irritation of a mixed nerve, it is sometimes found as a result of compression of a nerve or nerve root at a distance as in herniated lumbar disc and spinal cord tumor. (3) *Paralysis:* This is flaccid in nature and depends in degree on the amount of injury to the nerve. (4) *Atrophy:* Usually present but varies in degree; the principles governing the degree of atrophy in anterior horn cell disease hold true for peripheral nerves. (5) *Loss or diminution of reflexes.* (6) *Electromyographic evidence of denervation.* (7) *Sensory disturbances:* These appear in the appropriate peripheral nerve distribution, involving all types of sensation (pain, touch, heat, cold, position, vibration) in complete interruption and only superficial sensation in other cases (pain, touch, heat, cold). Hyperesthesia or paresthesias may occur.

LESIONS OF THE EXTRAPYRAMIDAL SYSTEM

The extrapyramidal system is a part of the motor apparatus composed of the basal ganglia and those portions of the cerebral cortex that have motor functions but are not part of the pyramidal or corticospinal system. There is controversy concerning precisely which subcortical nuclear masses should be included, but the following are generally agreed upon: caudate, putamen, pallidum, corpus subthalamicum, nucleus ruber, substantia nigra. Some include the thalamus and hypothalamus, as well as the cerebellum and the deep cerebellar, pontine, and olivary nuclei. All nuclei so included are richly connected with one another, but their precise functional interrelationships are not understood fully.

Disease of the extrapyramidal system results in disturbances of movement, as might be surmised from the motor function of the system. These are of three sorts: (1) akinetic or hypokinetic; (2) hyperkinetic; (3) mixed.

THE AKINETIC OR HYPOKINETIC SYNDROME

Paralysis agitans is typical of this, and may be used for illustrative purposes. Briefly, the parkinsonian patient characteristically exhibits muscular rigidity of cogwheeling type, which is elicited as follows: If the forearm is slowly pronated and supinated, or flexed and extended, the movement is felt as a series of catches and releases as if the muscle were being moved over a cog (hence the term cogwheel sign). Resistance tends to be uniform throughout the range of passive motion. There is marked poverty of movements, sometimes amounting to virtually complete immobility; the exact relationship of such akinetic phenomena to the muscular rigidity itself awaits clarification. Extreme difficulty in initiating movements is often found. Such movements as are carried out are generally slow, and few accessory movements are discerned. The head and trunk are held flexed, the face is fixed (so-called masked facies), and the speech is low and monotonous. A hyperkinetic element in the form of a resting tremor may also be present. Along with the reduced motility, slowing of mentation (bradyphrenia) is common, and, on occasion, true dementia appears. The tendon reflexes are usually normal and no Babinski sign is found.

HYPERKINETIC SYNDROMES

Choreiform Syndrome

This is seen most characteristically in the acute chorea of Sydenham and in the chronic progressive chorea of Huntington. It is evidenced by rapid, discrete, involuntary movements affecting the face and limbs, opposite muscle groups contracting simultaneously. Facial grimacing is common. Chorea is in all likelihood the result of disease of the caudate and perhaps of the corpus subthalamicum.

The choreiform movements are regarded as release phenomena, the cerebral cortex acting unopposed by the basal ganglia. Chorea is observed typically in degenerative disease of the striatum, as in Huntington's chorea; the pathological substrate of Sydenham's (rheumatic) chorea or chorea gravidarum is not definitely established. Choreiform movements have been reported on occasion with disease of many areas of the brain, including cortex, thalamus, red nucleus, and corpus subthalamicum. Chorea may be unilateral (hemichorea) and sufficiently violent to lead to confusion with the gross throwing or circling movements of the limbs, referred to as hemiballismus, that are observed with lesions in or near the corpus subthalamicum. A special variety of chorea, *posthemiplegic chorea,* may develop with recovery from hemiplegia in the affected limbs, as well as in the face; the occurrence of this syndrome under such circumstances has not been explained satisfactorily, though it is often attributed to residual sensory deficits.

Athetoid Syndrome

Athetoid movements are, in contrast to chorea, slow and sinuous movements composed of a mixture of irregularly synchronous contractions of opposite muscular groups (Wilson). They are most evident in the distal portions of the limbs, especially in the digits. Facial grimacing and movements of the head are common. Tongue movements are frequent, and speech and swallowing may be disturbed because of involvement of the pharyngeal muscles. The site of the lesion in cases of athetosis lies in the basal ganglia; although the exact areas involved are not definitely established, the pallidum and striatum appear the most likely candidates. As with chorea, the symptom of athetosis must be regarded as a release phenomenon. Separate ablation of the motor and premotor cortex results in permanent extinction of athetosis in some cases and temporary extinction in others; both chorea and athetosis tend to disappear after the spontaneous development of hemiplegia.

Pseudoathetosis is encountered with disease of the posterior columns, or dorsal roots, and reflects a loss of proprioception. It consists primarily of groping extensor movements of the fingers. Pseudoathetosis may appear in a variety of disorders, including tabes, syringomyelia, subacute combined degeneration, and multiple sclerosis.

Dystonic Syndrome

Even slower than athetoid movements are dystonic movements, which are slow, agonizing, writhing, virtually serpentine movements generally involving the proximal musculature of the limb girdles and of the neck and trunk; the movements sometimes seem to spread from the distal portion of the limbs to the proximal. The exact location of the lesions in the basal ganglia responsible for the appearance of dystonic movements is not clear, but the caudate and the putamen are most commonly implicated. This hyperkinetic disorder is seen in most striking form in that progressive familial disorder called dystonia musculorum deformans but may appear in a variety of other circumstances such as following carbon monoxide poisoning or as a residual of kernicterus. *Spasmodic torticollis* is sometimes looked upon as a fragmentary dystonic syndrome.

DISTURBANCES OF COORDINATION

The problem of coordination is a complex one. Three neural systems participate in the production of smooth coordinated movement: the posterior columns, the cerebellum, and the vestibular system. All are part of the proprioceptive system and all have important functions in the maintenance of posture: The vestibular system acts through the labyrinthine and righting reflexes; the posterior column, through the proprioceptors of muscles, tendons, and joints; and the cerebellum, through its action in synergizing movements. Impulses transmitted through the posterior column system reach consciousness, while those through the cerebellar pathway do not do so directly. The former may be regarded therefore as the conscious element of the proprioceptive system, and the latter, as its unconscious portion. Diseases of any of these systems results in disturbance of coordination, movement, and equilibrium.

Syndrome of the Posterior Column System

The posterior columns (gracilis and cuneatus) run the length of the spinal cord, the gracilis or column of Goll extending from the midthoracic cord downward and conveying impulses from the legs and lower trunk, and the cuneatus or column of Burdach extending from the midthoracic region upward and conveying impulses from the arms and upper trunk. The fibers from these columns decussate in the medulla, proceeding thence as the mesial fillet (or medial lemniscus) to the thalamus, whence they proceed to the cerebral cortex and particularly to the parietal lobe. They convey deep sensations from the muscles, joints, and tendons, measured clinically chiefly by position sense and vibration sense. Impulses conveyed through this system provide information regarding position of the limbs in space, and the force and range of movement. They provide one of the pathways for conveying touch sensation and two-point discrimination.

Diseases involving the posterior columns produce symptoms with the following characteristics: (1) They are dependent on sensory deficits, notably impairment or loss of muscle and position sense. By and large, the more severe this deficit, the more severe the symptoms. (2) They are the same regardless of location along the pathways from cord to cortex. The pattern in disease of the cerebral cortex is somewhat different. (3) Increase in symptoms follows elimination of vision. The degree of deficit, and, thus, of the resulting symptoms, depends on the severity and extent of the damage pathologically.

Ataxia is the outstanding symptom of lesions of the posterior column system. This ataxia is dependent on the loss of position sense and is increased by the shutting out of visual impulses. Thus, the ataxia of posterior column disease is

increased with the eyes closed, as in the Romberg test, and in the dark, as in
the gait disturbances of tabes or subacute combined degeneration. Patients with
posterior column disease consequently must watch the movements of the legs in
walking and of the arms in reaching. A characteristic feature of this form of
ataxia is the appearance of errors in range of movement, or *dysmetria*. Movements
such as putting the finger on the nose or the heel on the knee or toe overshoot
the mark, usually with gross irregularity of movement. Smooth coordinated movements become impossible. Dysmetria as seen under these circumstances reflects
inability to gauge the position of limbs in space and is thus dependent on sensory
(proprioceptive) deficit. Position sense is invariably lost or impaired in the
affected limbs, and the severity of the ataxia is usually in direct proportion to the
loss of position sense. It should of course be pointed out that loss of vibratory
sense alone, without concomitant loss of position sense, does not result in ataxia.

Though the symptoms resulting from deficit of proprioception are the *most*
striking evidences of posterior column disease, other symptoms are also found
associated with it but may not be as important clinically as ataxia. These consist
particularly of astereognosis and disturbance of two-point discrimination.

Posterior column disease occurs in a wide variety of conditions and of course
has the same clinical characteristics no matter what the pathological condition. It
is found in subacute combined degeneration, syringomyelia, multiple sclerosis,
spinal cord tumor, and a variety of other diseases; similar features may also appear
in disease of the posterior roots, such as tabes dorsalis. As already indicated, the
symptoms of posterior column affection are the same regardless of the point of

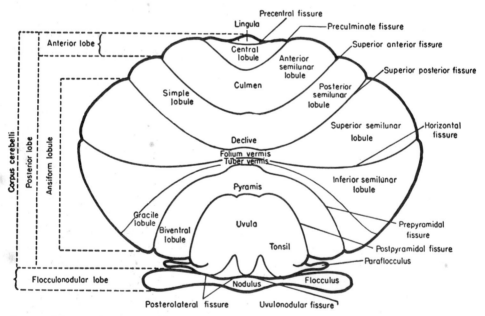

FIGURE 3-7. A diagram of the human cerebellum. (From Olaf Larsell: Anatomy of the
Nervous System, ed. 2, 1951. Courtesy of Appleton-Century-Crofts, Inc. Reproduced from
T. L. Peele's The Neuroanatomical Basis for Clinical Neurology.)

interruption of the system, whether in cervical or lumbar cord, in the mesial fillet in the brain stem, or in the thalamus.

Syndrome of the Cerebellar System

The cerebellum is intimately concerned with coordination of muscular contraction and maintenance of posture. It has very wide connections with all parts of the nervous system. It receives impulses from the trunk and limbs through the spinocerebellar pathways and from the head and neck probably through the external cuneate fibers. It is in intimate association with the vestibular system, basal ganglia and the tectum and has important though indirect connections with the cerebral cortex. A wide variety of nuclear aggregates of the brain stem, such as the olivary and arcuate nuclei, also exhibit significant relationships. The vast majority of these afferent fibers enter through the inferior and middle cerebellar peduncles (restiform body and brachium pontis). The principal efferent pathway is the superior cerebellar peduncle (brachium conjunctivum), carrying the dentatorubrothalamic fibers, which effect widespread connections in brain stem, basal ganglia, and cerebral cortex.

The basic symptom of deficit resulting from lesions of the cerebellum has been variously considered or interpreted as ataxia, defective maintenance of posture, asynergia, or hypotonia, or all of these. Regardless of the precise pathophysiological derangement, disease of the cerebellum regularly results in *loss or impairment of muscle coordination*, and the various signs that are encountered are expressions of this deficit. In a general way the clinical abnormalities found in cerebellar disease are ipsilateral, i.e., on the same side as the lesion.

A characteristic symptom of deficit of cerebellar disease is *asynergia* or *dyssynergia*. This consists of inability to perform movements smoothly because of the lack of normal synergistic action between the agonists and antagonists in muscle groups. The result is a jerky, highly incoordinate movement, a true decomposition of movement. The incoordination of cerebellar disease, unlike posterior column ataxia, has *no relation to vision* and is unaffected by eye closure or degree of illumination. More importantly, cerebellar asynergy is *not associated with sensory deficit,* and the disturbance of position and vibration senses found in posterior column ataxia is not found in cerebellar disease. In reaching for a goal, persons with cerebellar disease do so with intense incoordination and dysmetria, using accessory muscles of the arms or legs and describing a wide arc or trajectory. Unlike the individual with posterior column affection, however, they do reach the goal, though they may have difficulty in holding it. Thus, in placing the finger on the nose, a person with cerebellar disease will describe a wide arc with the arm, and with much jerking and tremor approach and finally reach the nose, whereas a patient with posterior column ataxia passes beyond it. Cerebellar dyssynergia is particularly well displayed in the cerebellar gait, generally described as ataxic in quality. It is performed on a wide base. The trunk and head are held stiffly, the legs shoot out from the hips, and the arms are flung about without relation to movement of the legs. There is considerable lurching and reeling. When dyssynergia involves the arms, the affected limbs droop slightly and drift outward on extension, and there is irregularity of movement in the patting test, in the rapid alternating or pronation-supination test, and in tests of manual dexterity.

Cerebellar disease is also characterized by *tremor*. This is present on voluntary movement of the limb (intention tremor) and is not evident with the limb at rest. It is a coarse oscillating tremor of wide amplitude, increasing in degree as the limb approaches the goal of its movement. It is seen more easily in the arms than in the legs.

Many patients with cerebellar disease exhibit *hypotonia* of the muscles and hypermotility at the joints. This is most evident in more acutely evolving cases. Some regard hypotonia as the essential and basic feature of cerebellar disease, responsible for faulty postural fixation, dyssynergia, tremor, etc. It may, however, be very difficult to demonstrate.

Cerebellar *speech* may be slow and hesitant, or completely dysarthric, probably as the result of asynergia of the musculature of the pharynx and larynx. Speech disturbances appear early in cerebellar disease and are often so slight as to be missed even by intelligent patients. A slight slowness and dragging of speech described as scanning characterizes the early stages.

Delay in starting and stopping muscle movement often occurs and is demonstrated by having the patient pull against resistance, the limb being suddenly released. The result is an *excessive rebound*, in which the patient may strike himself. The same phenomenon can be tested with the arms extended. Suddenly pushing down on the affected arm results in a pendular response. Excessive rebound undoubtedly reflects faulty postural fixation; the same mechanism accounts for the *pendular reflexes*, best seen with the patellar reflexes. *Loss of*

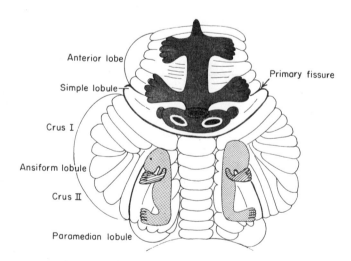

FIGURE 3-8. Somatotopic localization in the cerebellar cortex, based on the results of numerous animal studies and confirmed to at least some extent in man. The representation on the superior face (anterior lobe, simple lobule) appears of greatest clinical significance. (Modified from Snider, R. S.: Interrelations of Cerebellum and Brain Stem. Res. Publ. Assoc. Res. Nerv. Ment. Dis. 30:267, 1952.)

ASYNERGIA
1. DYSMETRIA
2. ANP.O-MPOELNANDE
3. GAIT DISTURBANCE

associated movement such as swinging the arm in walking may also be seen in cerebellar disease.

Cerebellar symptoms when pronounced are easily recognized but require experience to evaluate in minor degrees. They may be recognized by the presence of asynergia, by the various tests described earlier, by observation of the typical gait, and by tremor, hypotonia, and dysarthria. In pronounced cases most or all of these features will be present. Severe tremor may on occasion be found with little or no asynergia, or asynergia may be found with only minimal tremor. It is, further, essential to recognize that cerebellar signs may involve the trunk without involvement of the limbs, or vice versa. As in the cerebral cortex, so too in the cerebellar cortex a pattern of somatotopic localization can be defined, and focal lesions will give rise to affection of the trunk or of the limbs, depending on their exact location. The trunk appears represented in the midline (vermis), especially superiorly, the limbs more laterally in the hemispheres; the legs seem represented anteriorly and superiorly, the arms posteriorly and superiorly. Thus, lesions in the vermis are associated with truncal incoordination and ataxia, whereas lesions in the hemispheres give rise predominantly to incoordination of the appropriate (ipsilateral) limbs.

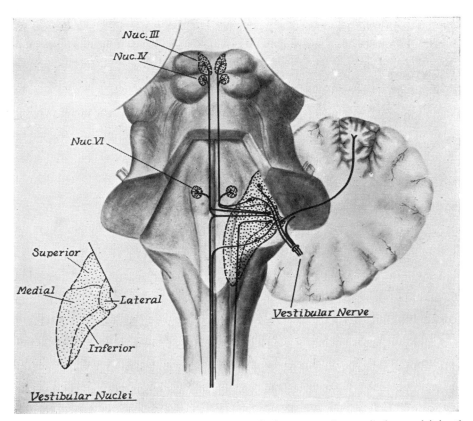

FIGURE 3-9. Vestibular system, showing the vestibular nerve, the vestibular nuclei in the medulla, and their connections in the brain stem.

Generally speaking, the symptoms of cerebellar disease are the same regardless of the point of interruption of the cerebellar apparatus, and it may not be possible to distinguish affection of the cerebellum itself from that of its pathways and tracts. Tremor, however, is most pronounced with involvement of the superior cerebellar peduncle, becoming increasingly prominent as the lesion approaches the red nucleus.

Syndrome of the Vestibular System

Disturbances of the vestibular system may result from lesions in the labyrinths, the vestibular nerve, the vestibular pathways within the brain stem, the cerebrum, or cerebellum. The anatomy of the vestibular fibers is complex. Fibers pass from the labyrinth to the vestibular nerve, which forms part of the auditory nerve, and are distributed to the vestibular nuclei in the medulla. From this point, impulses descend to end around anterior horn cells in the spinal cord, or ascend with or without synapse into the cerebellum. Significant connections are also made with the posterior longitudinal bundle, ending in the oculomotor nuclei, both crossed and uncrossed, and the reticular formation.

Interruption of the vestibular system results in the production of *vertigo,* a purely subjective sensation characterized by a disturbance of equilibrium resulting from illusory movement of the individual or his surroundings. *Nausea* and *vomiting* commonly accompany vertigo, particularly in acute instances. *Nystagmus* (see Chapter 2) is frequent; it may be horizontal, vertical, or rotary, the latter being especially prominent when the lesion involves the labyrinth itself. *Ataxia* or incoordination is often striking with vestibular disease; it can generally be distinguished from cerebellar ataxia by virtue of the associated vertigo.

LESIONS INVOLVING SUPERFICIAL SENSATION

Deep sensation has already been dealt with. It remains to consider the disturbances of superficial sensation occurring at various levels of the nervous system. These may involve: (1) spinal roots; (2) peripheral nerve; (3) spinal cord (commissure, tract, hemisection, and complete transverse syndromes); (4) brain stem; (5) thalamus, and (6) cerebral cortex.

Root Syndrome

The posterior roots entering the spinal cord may be involved in a variety of diseases, such as tabes dorsalis, herpes zoster, spinal cord tumor, metastatic carcinoma, pachymeningitis, tuberculosis of the spine, herniated intervertebral disc, and a host of other conditions. The posterior root syndrome is characterized by (a) *Pain.* The pain of this syndrome is referred along the specific roots as shown in Figure 3-10. It is severe, constant or intermittent, often lancinating in quality, and radiates along the root or roots affected. It is usually increased on coughing, straining, sneezing, or with any maneuver that increases intraspinal pressure.

Increase of pain in this fashion probably results from sudden distention with spinal fluid of the subarachnoid sheath surrounding the root, with irritation or compression of the affected root by the sudden wave of fluid. While increase with cough and strain indicates root pain, its absence does not exclude it. Although root pain is almost always severe, it may actually be unbearable, particularly in cases of acute radiculitis of inflammatory origin. (b) *Sensory disturbances.* These may be in the nature of hyperesthesia in irritative lesions, or of loss of superficial sensation (touch, pain, temperature) in the appropriate root distribution. Since there is much overlapping of adjacent roots it is often difficult to map out sensory defects in root disturbances unless they are multiple.

Peripheral Nerve Syndrome

The full syndrome has been discussed under the section of the lower motor neuron. The sensory disturbances in lesions of the peripheral nerve are characterized by: (1) complete loss of all forms of sensation (touch, pain, heat, cold, position, vibration) in complete interruption of the nerve; (2) partial loss of sensation in incomplete lesions. These sensory disturbances are found in the

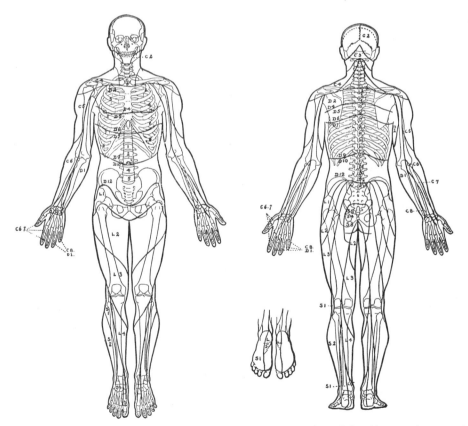

FIGURE 3-10. Root sensory skin innervation. A diagrammatic view of the skin areas innervated by the posterior roots.

distribution of the peripheral nerve which of course differs from that of the roots. In a typical mononeuropathy, or mononeuritis, therefore, the sensory impairment follows a distribution predictable from knowledge of the anatomy of the particular nerve involved. In the more common polyneuropathies, the alteration of sensation tends to assume a glove and stocking pattern, reflecting the affection of the distal twigs of a number of sensory nerves.

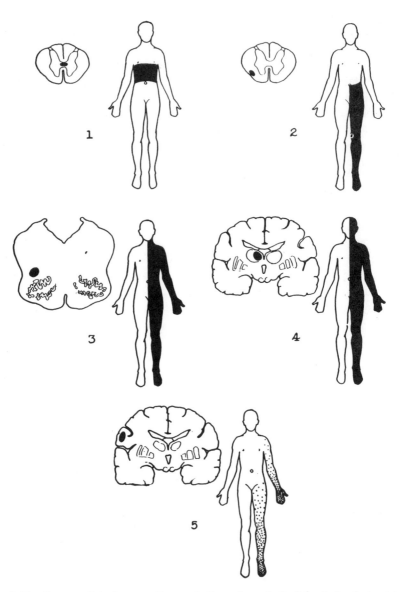

FIGURE 3-11.   Sensory disturbance patterns. 1. Commissural. 2. Spinothalamic tract in cord. 3. Spinothalamic tract in medulla. 4. Thalamus. 5. Sensory cortex.

Spinal Cord Syndrome

COMMISSURAL SYNDROME.   This is the result of a lesion involving the central gray matter of the spinal cord. It is found particularly in syringomyelia but may be found also in trauma (hematomyelia), syphilitic meningomyelitis, spinal cord tumor, and other conditions. It is characterized by a loss of pain and temperature sensation due to the interruption of these fibers as they cross to the spinothalamic tract. The sensory loss is bilateral, since fibers from both sides must inevitably be interrupted in such a lesion, and segmental, involving only the fibers of the segments involved. Thus, a lesion involving the central gray matter of segments T2 to T5 will produce loss of pain and temperature sensation only in these segments. The commissural syndrome can be produced only by a lesion within the cord substance. It is anatomically impossible for an extramedullary lesion to produce the syndrome.

POSTERIOR HORN SYNDROME.   Ipsilateral impairment of pain and temperature may be found with involvement of the pain and temperature fibers in the posterior horn before they decussate in the commissure. This is usually the result of a slitlike syringomyelic cavity, and the resulting sensory disturbance may extend for a variable number of segments. If the lesion extends into the root entry zone, radicular pain may also appear.

SPINOTHALAMIC TRACT SYNDROME.   A lesion involving the spinothalamic tract in the anterolateral portion of the spinal cord causes a loss of pain and temperature sensations on the opposite side of the body, involving all the segments below the level of the lesion. Pain and temperature sensations may not be involved with equal severity; one, usually pain, may be affected more than the other. A variety of both intramedullary and extramedullary processes may give rise to the syndrome. Within the spinothalamic tract the fibers are arranged in

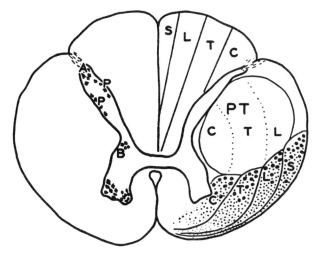

FIGURE 3-12. Spinal cord. Diagrammatic arrangement of the fibers of the spinothalamic tract is clearly shown, the sacral fibers being at the outer edge. (After Walker.)

laminar fashion, the sacral fibers being located at the periphery, fibers from higher levels more centrally. Hence, an intramedullary process will involve the fibers from the higher levels first and often spare the sacral fibers. This is referred to as *sacral sparing* and is commonly although not invariably observed with intramedullary processes. Extramedullary processes, on the other hand, compress the cord from without and result in involvement of the sacral fibers as well as those from higher levels. It will incidentally be noted that a reverse lamellation obtains in the posterior columns, the lumbar and sacral fibers being found most deeply, the cervical most laterally.

BROWN-SÉQUARD SYNDROME. This is seen in its purest form in hemisection of the spinal cord. It consists of:

On the side of the lesion: Paralysis, loss of position and vibration senses, and ataxia.

On the side opposite the lesion: Loss of pain and temperature senses.

This syndrome, which may result from both intramedullary and extramedullary lesions, is not usually seen in complete form. It more commonly presents in incomplete or impure fashion, usually as loss of pain and temperature senses on the opposite side of the body below the level of the lesion, with but few ipsilateral signs.

COMPLETE TRANSVERSE SYNDROME. This syndrome is of great importance and should be clearly recognized. It is found in many conditions, including trauma, spinal cord tumor, metastatic tumor, spinal cord syphilis, multiple sclerosis, and acute disseminated encephalomyelitis. It is characterized by:

Paralysis below the level of the lesion.

Complete *loss of all modalities of sensation* below the level of the lesion. In some instances, especially extramedullary cord tumors, there is a zone of hyperesthesia at the top of the level.

Sphincter disturbances. There is retention of urine in acute cases, which in the course of a few days or weeks develops into automatic emptying. Fecal incontinence is found in complete interruption.

Trophic disturbances. These are manifested by trophic ulcers of the skin, disturbances of the nails, etc. A loss of sweating is generally found below the level of the lesion as well.

The manifestations of transverse lesions of the spinal cord vary with the rapidity of development of the process. In acutely developing transverse sections as seen in cord injuries, myelitis, etc., the manifestations are those of *spinal shock*. The paralyzed muscles are toneless and flaccid, the superficial and tendon reflexes are absent, there is complete sensory loss below the level of the lesion, and retention of urine and feces is found. This stage may last 3 weeks or longer and is then followed by a phase of recovery of reflex activity. This is manifested by a return of flexor reflexes in response to noxious stimuli applied to the skin, at times with a *mass reflex* characterized by flexor spasm of the legs and lower abdominal wall, evacuation of the bladder, and sweating. The tendon reflexes return during this stage and are exaggerated. Reflex emptying of the bladder and bowel may also appear at this time.

With more gradually evolving transverse lesions such as intramedullary tumor, spinal shock is not encountered. The legs become weak and spastic, and eventually completely paralyzed if the process is not relieved. Weakness usually develops before sensory loss in cases of compression from without, as in extramedullary tumors, since motor fibers appear more susceptible than sensory to injury. Gradually, however, sensory impairment also ensues. Alterations in sphincter control generally parallel the appearance of pyramidal tract signs. The final result is a transverse syndrome characterized by spastic paraplegia, sensory loss, and sphincter abnormalities.

Thalamic Syndrome

The thalamus is the end station of all crude forms of sensibility. A complete lesion of the thalamus will cause: (1) loss of all forms of sensation involving the opposite side of the face, trunk, and limbs; (2) astereognosis; (3) central pains on the opposite side; these may be deep, paroxysmal, and excruciating in nature, but not uncommonly are burning and causalgia-like. They may involve the entire side of the body or be confined to portions of it. Pain stimuli cause unpleasant sensations, often with radiation of the pain beyond the point of stimulation. Hot, cold, and tactile stimuli may cause the same type of over-reaction as pain. The combination of sensory loss, spontaneous pain, and perversion of cutaneous sensibility (dysesthesias) is sometimes referred to as the thalamic syndrome of Déjerine-Roussy. The impairment of sensation may be relatively mild as compared to the degree of spontaneous pain.

Cortical Syndrome

Sensory disturbances due to involvement of the sensory parietal cortex are not as sharply defined as in lesions involving lower levels. Discriminatory sensations are more severely affected than superficial or crude sensations. In general, one observes: (1) Loss of position sense. Vibration sense may or may not be involved. Some investigators deny the involvement of vibration sense in lesions confined to the sensory cortex. (2) Absence of consistent involvement of other crude forms of sensation, such as pain, touch, and temperature. Pain sensation may, however, be decreased, particularly in distal portions of the limbs. Touch, heat, and cold are not usually affected. Spontaneous pain has been reported in tumors and cysts of the sensory cortex. (3) Impairment of discrimination as, for example, detecting the two points of a compass, appreciating differences in texture, recognizing figures written on the skin, and appreciating differences in weight. These elements are the most severely affected in cortical lesions. (4) Astereognosis, or the inability to recognize the shape or nature of objects placed in the hand. The problem of astereognosis is complex, and much remains to be elucidated. Stereognosis is the ability to recognize the size, shape, weight, and other physical characteristics of objects and is dependent upon the capacity to synthesize these individual characteristics into a meaningful whole (gestalt). A loss of this ability is called astereognosis, or "tactile agnosia." It is regarded by some as dependent on sensory disturbances, particularly loss of touch and proprioception, but this is not universally accepted, and there are those who believe that it is not possible to speak of astereognosis unless there is intact sensation. (5) Sensory jacksonian seizures.

The parietal lobe syndrome is also characterized by the occurrence of agnosia (see below). In addition, with rapidly evolving lesions such as softenings involving the minor parietal lobe, disturbances of the body scheme (see above) appear. There is disagreement as to whether the body image is in fact localized to the nondominant parietal lobe, or whether it is bilaterally represented. According to the latter view, the presence of language disorders (aphasia) with dominant hemispheral lesions precludes evaluation of the body image in the majority of cases and leads to an erroneous impression of lateralization of function.

LESIONS OF SPHINCTERS

Loss of sphincter control occurs under many circumstances in the human. The problem is complex, and a review of the normal control of the sphincters is pertinent. Disturbances of micturition are of greater practical significance than those of defecation and are much more frequent.

Bladder

The bladder empties by means of a reciprocal action of its involuntary musculature, the detrusor, and the internal sphincter. These receive their innervation through the hypogastric (T11, T12, and L1) and sacral nerves, the former derived from the lumbar sympathetic chain, the latter from the sacral plexus by the pelvic nerves (S2, 3, 4). The external sphincter and the voluntary muscles of the perineum are innervated by the pudendal nerves (S2, 3, 4). The parasympathetic center for micturition in the spinal cord is in segments S2 and S3, the sympathetic center lying in the lumbar cord.

Stimulation of the peripheral segment of the cut pelvic nerves in animals causes powerful contraction of the detrusor muscle with relaxation of the internal sphincter. Stimulation of the hypogastric nerves causes contraction of the internal sphincter in animals and man, accompanied by inhibition of action of the detrusor. Stimulation of the pudendal nerve causes contraction of the external sphincter. The integrity of the pelvic nerves is of paramount importance for normal micturition; section of these nerves causes profound depression of micturition with an atonic distended bladder. Section of the hypogastric, pelvic, and pudendal nerves is followed, after a short period of retention, by periodic discharge or automatic micturition.

Control of the bladder musculature for the reflex act of micturition is effected by cerebral mechanisms as well as by those at the spinal cord level. Cerebral control of the bladder seems to be inhibitory in function since removal of the motor cortex in animals either unilaterally or bilaterally results in overaction of the reflex of micturition. Stimulation of this area results in bladder contraction and emptying. The cortical area responsible for bladder control lies near the leg area of the motor cortex; in man, lesions of the paracentral lobule result in incontinence.

The normal act of micturition is dependent on a stretch reflex acting on the detrusor muscle, the stimulus being the stretch evoked by the increasing volume of the bladder contents and by the resultant rise in intravesical pressure. As a result of distention of the bladder, afferent impulses reach the spinal cord, the detrusor contracts as the result of impulses conveyed through the pelvic nerves, and reciprocal relaxation of the sphincter follows.

TYPES OF BLADDER DISTURBANCE. Two main types are found in the human, *atonic* and *hypertonic*. The unfortunate term "neurogenic" or "cord" bladder has arisen to designate bladder disturbances of peripheral or central nervous system origin. The term is meaningless, and whenever possible the precise form of bladder dysfunction should be designated. The *atonic bladder* is found particularly in lesions of the sacral segments of the spinal cord (conus medullaris) and in diseases of the cauda equina and pelvic nerves. It is characterized by atonic bladder musculature due to loss of tone of the detrusor muscle, increased bladder capacity, and loss of sensation associated with bladder distention, so that the patient is unable to tell when the bladder is full. The bladder under such circumstances may become very large and may actually reach to the umbilicus without a sensation of distention. Destructive lesions of the sacral cord or its roots are

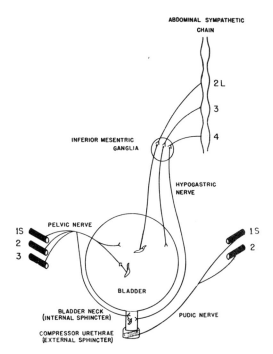

FIGURE 3-13. Innervations of bladder, showing the central and peripheral innervations of the detrusor, and the internal and external sphincters. (From Learmonth & McLeod: Physiology in Modern Medicine, 9th ed., p. 1128, C. V. Mosby Co.)

followed, therefore, by retention of urine with distention of the bladder. This is followed by automatic emptying of the bladder, which, however, almost never empties completely. Urine in such cases is discharged in small amounts at a time; in some instances complete emptying may occur. The cystometrogram in such cases reveals increased bladder capacity, a very slow rise in the vesical pressure during filling, and the ability to retain a large amount of fluid before sufficient stretch is produced to cause reflex contraction of the bladder.

An atonic bladder response is also found in lesions involving the posterior roots of the spinal cord or the posterior columns, lesions that interfere with the afferent side of the reflex arc. This occurs in particularly striking fashion in tabes dorsalis. In this form of atonic bladder, the bladder capacity is also greatly increased, there is no sensation of distention of the bladder, the detrusor tone is lost, and there is incontinence due to relaxation of the internal sphincter and impaired detrusor action. Emptying the bladder is possible by normal volition, but the stream is feeble and residual urine is always found.

The atonic bladder thus results essentially from interruption of the afferent or efferent peripheral pathways to the bladder, or both. In contrast is the *hypertonic bladder,* which results from interruption of the central pathways. This may result from lesions of the spinal cord, usually bilateral, anywhere above the sacral segments, or from involvement of the motor cortex or of the pyramidal tract anywhere along its course. In the hypertonic bladder, capacity is reduced, in contrast to the distended atonic bladder. The vesical pressure rises rapidly during filling, so that relatively little urine can collect before the desire for micturition develops. Urgency and frequency are thus characteristic. Unlike the atonic bladder, sensation is not lost and bladder distention is associated with a feeling of discomfort. The bladder is emptied completely with each act of urination.

An *automatic bladder* may become established in instances of complete transection of the cord above the sacral segments. Following the stage of paralysis and distention of the bladder automatic contraction of the bladder wall develops with expulsion of urine but without complete emptying of the bladder. At times the automatic emptying is part of the mass reflex already described. Automatic bladder function may develop in 4 to 5 weeks after cord transection, but in many instances it fails to develop, a fact that must be given due consideration in the treatment of transverse cord lesions.

Rectum

The normal act of defecation is characterized by contraction of the rectum and reciprocal relaxation of the anal sphincter. The adequate stimulus is tension on the wall of the rectum, which brings about a stretch reflex and contraction of the rectum. The reciprocal relationship between rectum and internal sphincter is nervous in mechanism and is mediated solely through the lower sacral segments of the spinal cord (S2, 3, 4) and its peripheral plexuses. Destruction of the sacral segments of the spinal cord or its roots results in relaxation of the sphincter and continuous bowel evacuation, whereas destruction of the cord above the sacral segments causes intermittent involuntary emptying of the bowel.

BIBLIOGRAPHY

Alpers, B. J., and Mancall, E. L.: Chapter 31, in Sodeman, W. A., and Sodeman, W. A., Jr. (eds.): Pathologic Physiology: Mechanisms of Disease, ed. 4. W. B. Saunders Co., Philadelphia, 1967.

Bender, M. B., and Bergman, P. S.: Neuroophthalmology (Nystagmus). Progr. Neurol. Psychiat. 10:201, 1955.

Brain, L.: Speech Disorders: Aphasia, Apraxia, and Agnosia. Butterworths, Washington, 1965.

Brock, S. A.: Basis of Clinical Neurology, ed. 3. Williams & Wilkins Co., Baltimore, 1953.

Brown, J. R.: Localizing Cerebellar Symptoms. J.A.M.A. 141: 518, 1949.

Chambers, W. W., and Sprague, J. M.: Functional Localization in the Cerebellum. II. Somatotopic Organization of Cortex and Nuclei. Arch. Neurol Psychiat. 74:6, 1955.

Chapman, L. F., and Wolff, H. G.: Cerebral Hemispheres and Highest Integrative Functions of Man. Arch. Neurol. Psychiat. 1:357, 1959.

Cogan, D.: Neurology of the Ocular Muscles, ed. 2. Charles C Thomas, Springfield, Ill., 1963.

Cogan, D. G.: Neurology of the Visual System. Charles C Thomas, Springfield, Ill., 1966.

Critchley, M.: Developmental Dyslexia. William Heinemann, London, 1964.

Critchley, M.: The Parietal Lobes. Hafner Publishing Co., New York, 1953.

Darley, F. L., and Millikan, C. H. (eds.): Brain Mechanisms Underlying Speech and Language. Grune & Stratton, New York, 1967.

DeJong, R. N.: Nystagmus: An Appraisal and Classification. Arch. Neurol. Psychiat. 55:43, 1946.

Denny-Brown, D.: Diseases of the Basal Ganglia: Their Relation to Disorders of Movement. Lancet 2:1099, 1155, 1960.

Denny-Brown, D., and Robertson, E. G.: On the Physiology of Micturition. Brain 56:149, 1933.

Denny-Brown, D., and Robertson, E. G.: An Investigation of the Nervous Control of Defecation. Brain 58:256, 1935.

Disorders of Communication (Rioch, D. McK., and Weinstein, E. A. (eds.)). Res. Publ. Assoc. Res. Nerv. Ment. Dis., volume 42, 1964.

Dow, R. S.: Effect of Lesions in the Vestibular Part of the Cerebellum in Primates. Arch. Neurol. Psychiat. 40:500, 1938.

Dow, R. S., and Moruzzi, G.: The Physiology and Pathology of the Cerebellum. University of Minnesota Press, Minneapolis, 1958.

Ettlinger, E. G., deReuck, A. V. S., and Porter, R. (eds.): Functions of the Corpus Callosum, Ciba Foundation Study Group No. 20. Little, Brown and Co., Boston, 1965.

Ferraro, A., and Barrera, S. E.: Effects of Experimental Lesions of the Posterior Columns in Macacus Rhesus Monkeys. Brain 57:307, 1934.

Ferraro, A., and Barrera, S. E.: The Posterior Column Nuclei in Macacus Rhesus Monkeys. Arch. Neurol. Psychiat. 32:434, 1934.

Ferraro, A., Barrera, S. E., and Blakeslee, G. A.: Vestibular Phenomena of Central Origin. Brain 59:466, 1936.

Fischer, J. J.: The Labyrinth—Physiology and Functional Tests. Grune & Stratton, New York, 1956.

Fox, J. C., and Holmes, G.: Optic Nystagmus and Its Value in the Localization of Cerebral Lesions. Brain 49:333, 1926.

Geschwind, N.: Disconnexion Syndromes in Animals and Man. Brain 88:237, 585, 1965.

Geschwind, N.: The Clinical Syndromes of the Cortical Connections, Chapter 2 in Williams, D. (ed.): Modern Trends in Neurology. Butterworths, London, 1970.

Geschwind, N.: Aphasia. New Eng. J. Med. 284:654, 1971.

Goldstein, K.: Language and Language Disturbances. Grune & Stratton, New York, 1948.

Gorman, W. F., and Brock, S.: Nystagmus: Its Mechanism and Significance. Amer. J. Med. Sci. 220:225, 1950.

Head, H.: Aphasia and Kindred Disorders of Speech. Macmillan Co., New York, 1926.

Hines, M.: Control of Movements by the Cerebral Cortex in Primates. Biol. Rev. 18:1, 1943.

Jung, R., and Hassler, R.: The Extrapyramidal Motor System, in Handbook of Physiology. American Physiological Society, Washington, 1960. Section I: Neurophysiology, vol. 2, p. 863.

Langworthy, O. R., and Kolb, L. C.: The Encephalic Control of Tone in the Musculature of the Urinary Bladder. Brain 56:371, 1933.

Luria, A. R.: The Role of Speech in the Regulation of Normal and Abnormal Behavior. Liveright Publishing Corp., New York, 1961.

Luria, A. R.: Human Brain and Psychological Processes. Harper & Row, New York, 1966.

Magoun, H., and Rhines, R.: Spasticity. Charles C Thomas. Springfield, Ill., 1947.

McNally, W. J., and Stuart, E. A.: Chapter I, in Ellis, M. (ed.): Modern Trends in Diseases of the Ear, Nose and Throat. Paul B. Hoeber, New York, 1954.

Meyjes, F. P.: The Localization and Pathophysiology of the Choreatic Movement. Ztschr. ges. Neur. u. Psychiat. 133:1, 1931.

Moruzzi, G.: Problems in Cerebellar Physiology. Charles C Thomas, Springfield, Ill., 1950.

Monrad-Krohm, G. H.: Clinical Examination of the Nervous System, ed. 11. Paul B. Hoeber, New York, 1958.

Nielsen, J. M.: Agnosia, Apraxia, Aphasia: Their Value in Cerebral Localization. Paul B. Hoeber, New York, 1946.

Nylen, C. O.: Positional Nystagmus. J. Laryng. 64:295, 1950.

Osgood, C., and Miron, M.: Approaches to the Study of Aphasia. University of Illinois Press, Urbana, Ill., 1963.

Peele, T. L.: Neuroanatomical Basis of Clinical Neurology. McGraw-Hill Book Co., New York, 1954.

Penfield, W.: The Cerebral Cortex in Man. I. The Cerebral Cortex and Consciousness. Arch. Neurol. Psychiat. 40:417, 1938.

Penfield, W., and Roberts, L.: Speech and Brain-Mechanisms. Princeton University Press, Princeton, N. J., 1959.

Purves-Stewart, J., and Worster-Drought, C.: Diagnosis of Nervous Diseases, ed. 10. Williams & Wilkins Co., Baltimore, 1952.

Spiegel, E. A., and Sommer, I.: Vestibular Mechanisms, in Glasser, O. (ed.): Medical Physics. Year Book Publishers, Chicago, 1944.

Terzuolo, C. A., and Adey, W. R.: Sensorimotor Cortical Activities, in Handbook of Physiology. American Physiological Society, Washington, 1960. Section I: Neurophysiology, vol. 2, pp. 797-836.

von Bonin, G.: Some Papers on the Cerebral Cortex. Charles C Thomas, Springfield, Ill., 1960.

Walshe, F. M. R.: Cortical Studies in Neurology. Williams & Wilkins Co., Baltimore, 1948.

Weisenburg, T., and McBride, K. E.: Aphasia: A Clinical and Psychological Study (1935). Hafner Publishing Co., New York, 1964 (reprint).

Wepman, J. M., and Jones, L. V.: Five Aphasias: A Commentary on Aphasia as a Regressive Linguistic Phenomenon. Res. Publ. Assoc. Res. Nerv. Ment. Dis. 42:190, 1964.

Wilson, S. A. K.: Disorders of Motility and Muscle Tone, with Special Reference to Corpus Striatum. Lancet 2:1, 53, 169, 215, 1925.

Wilson, S. A. K.: Aphasia. Psyche Miniatures—Medical Series No. 2. Paul Kegan, London, 1926.

CHAPTER 4

Laboratory Investigations in Neurological Disease

Since a variety of special examinations is often required in the study of diseases of the nervous system, brief consideration of some of the more common techniques employed, and of the results obtained, seems appropriate.

LUMBAR PUNCTURE

Lumbar puncture, and detailed examination of the cerebrospinal fluid obtained thereby, represents in many ways the simplest as well as the most informative of the ancillary tests available to the clinical neurologist. It should be performed, however, only with the greatest caution in the presence of increased intracranial pressure, and it is particularly hazardous in instances of expanding lesions in the posterior fossa. The risk of herniation of the brain under pressure through either the free edge of the tentorium (uncal herniation) or foramen magnum (cerebellar tonsillar herniation) should not be underestimated under these circumstances; even if only a small amount of spinal fluid is removed at the time of the tap, continued leakage of fluid through the puncture wound in the meninges may lead to delayed herniation. In general, lumbar puncture must be carried out in the presence of an increase in intracranial pressure only when absolutely necessary for diagnostic purposes, as, for example, when the possibility of purulent meningitis must be excluded, and then only with full knowledge of the risks being undertaken.

Proper position of the patient is essential for a good lumbar puncture. The patient is placed on his side on a hard surface such as a stretcher, or is brought to the edge of the bed. The subject must lie squarely on the bed. The head and body should be acutely flexed, the knees being drawn up on the abdomen and clasped firmly by the hands. The back is prepared with iodine and 70 per cent alcohol, or other cutaneous antiseptics. Sterile towels should be placed under the back and over the buttocks; alternatively, a surgical drape may be used.

The puncture should be performed under aseptic precautions, with sterile gloves. The needle should be sharp and as small as consistent with accurate pressure readings. The tap is best made between the fourth and fifth or third and fourth lumbar vertebrae, the latter being preferred because of frequent anomalies involving the former. The level utilized is estimated by palpating the iliac crest, which ordinarily lies opposite the fourth lumbar vertebra.

Procaine is injected into the skin as a local anesthetic. The lumbar puncture needle may be inserted in the midline or about 1 cm. to one side of the midline and is directed slightly upward. Entrance into the subarachnoid space is felt as a "give" before the needle as it penetrates the dura, the subarachnoid membrane lying immediately below it. If the puncture has been performed without trauma, clear fluid is obtained on withdrawal of the stylet. The manometer for measuring pressure of the spinal fluid should be attached at this point without loss of any of the spinal fluid. A water manometer is preferable, but a mercury manometer may be used. The level of the fluid column should be measured after it has come to rest. If the patient is tense this may require 4 or 5 minutes or longer; if he is relaxed an accurate pressure reading may be taken within this time.

In cases of suspected block of the spinal subarachnoid space a so-called Queckenstedt test may be performed. It should never be performed in instances of disease above the foramen magnum, especially if a brain tumor is suspected. The test is performed with the aid of an assistant, who compresses one jugular vein for 10 seconds, then the other, and then both simultaneously; a blood pressure cuff may also be utilized to exert pressure evenly. The rise of pressure at the end of 10 seconds is recorded; the compression is then released, and the level of pressure recorded 10 seconds later. In normal persons with no block of the subarachnoid space when the spinal needle is well placed, a rapid and high rise of spinal fluid pressure (to 400 or 500 mm. of water) follows bilateral jugular compression. Return of the pressure to its original level takes place in 10 to 15 seconds after release of the pressure. The test is completed by having the patient strain, then cough; a similar rise in pressure occurs. The elevation of intraspinal pressure following compression of the jugular veins is due to increase in intracranial pressure as a result of interference with venous escape from the skull. If a block is present in the subarachnoid space, no rise, or only an imperfect one, occurs with jugular compression. Coughing and straining will still elicit a rise in pressure, however, because the increased abdominal pressure prevents escape of blood from the spinal veins.

After the dynamic examination is completed, fluid is removed for routine examination, which should consist of determination of cell count, protein and sugar content, colloidal gold reaction, and appropriate tests for syphilis. Special studies, such as smear and culture or estimation of the gamma globulin, should

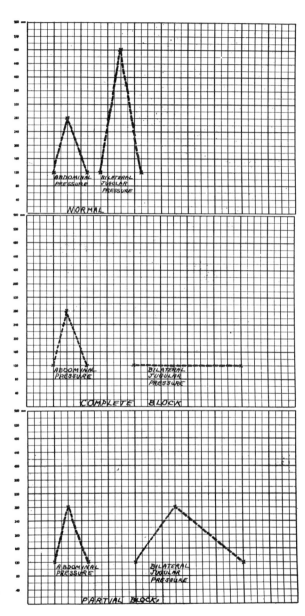

FIGURE 4-1. Subarachnoid block shown in diagrammatic form. In top panel is shown the rapid rise and fall of spinal fluid pressure on abdominal straining and bilateral jugular compression. In the middle panel is shown a failure of increase of spinal fluid pressure with complete block. In the lower panel is shown the delayed rise and fall of spinal fluid pressure on jugular compression in partial subarachnoid block.

be made as indicated. The level of the spinal fluid pressure is recorded routinely after the fluid is withdrawn. The spinal fluid, particularly if bloody, should be drawn into several successive tubes. This technique is especially valuable in the identification of a traumatic tap, the blood under such a circumstance generally disappearing by the third tube.

The puncture wound is covered with a sterile dressing and the patient instructed to lie flat, but not necessarily on his back, for 8 to 24 hours in order to avoid a lumbar puncture headache. The diet after puncture needs no restrictions; the intake of liquids should be encouraged.

Cistern Puncture

This is necessary only under exceptional circumstances and should be avoided if at all possible because of its inherent risks. The hair should be shaved to the level of the occipital protuberances. The patient is placed on his side, with the head sharply flexed, the chin on the chest, and the head absolutely straight. Rotation of the neck must be avoided. The back of the neck is prepared with iodine and alcohol and the head and shoulders draped with sterile towels. The puncture itself is performed with aseptic precautions, a lumbar puncture needle being used.

The spine of the second cervical vertebra is identified and the thumb of the examiner's left hand is held firmly down on this spine. The needle is then directed along the knuckle of the flexed left thumb, the point coming directly in the center of the depression above the second cervical spine. The needle is then directed in the midline slightly upward along a line transecting the external auditory meatus and the bridge of the nose. After two or three resistances are encountered a sudden "give" is felt, indicating entrance of the needle into the cisterna magna. This is reached in thin-necked persons at a depth of about 4 cm., and in thick-necked persons, at about 5 cm. If blood is encountered the needle should be withdrawn and no further attempts made. If the neck has been in good position, and the needle held strictly in the midline in the direction indicated, the cistern will be reached without difficulty.

The Cerebrospinal Fluid

The *normal* spinal fluid pressure as recorded at lumbar puncture utilizing a water manometer varies from 100 to 200 mm. Pressures over 200 mm. are definitely elevated; those of 190 to 200 mm. are borderline. The cell content of the spinal fluid varies normally from one to six lymphocytes; a cell content of ten cells or more is abnormal. The spinal fluid normally has a protein content of 25 to 45 mg. per 100 ml. Globulin is present in slight amounts. The sugar content varies from 50 to 80 mg. per 100 ml., the precise level being determined by the concentration in the blood. The Wassermann reaction and other tests for syphilis are, of course, negative. In some instances the chloride content is sought; this ranges normally from 725 to 750 mg. The colloidal gold test, often looked upon as an indirect measure of gamma globulin content, is read normally as follows: 0000000000 (0^{10}). Direct measurement of gamma globulin ordinarily yields a level under 12 per cent.

Smear and culture of the spinal fluid are indicated in instances of nervous system infection and must be done before antimicrobial therapy is instituted. Bacteria may be demonstrated by smear in many infections of the meninges but on occasion are found only with great difficulty; tubercle bacilli are particularly elusive. Viruses are of course not found in this fashion. Parasites, yeasts, and fungi may be found on smear in rare cases but may require special staining techniques, as, for example, India ink in instances of torulosis.

Abnormalities of the spinal fluid are found under many circumstances; a search for such variations constitutes one of the most important aspects of investigation of disease of the nervous system.

PRESSURE. Disturbances of cerebrospinal fluid pressure are found in many conditions. Increased pressure is found in (1) brain tumor, though not invariably. It is practically always elevated in posterior fossa tumors, especially those involving the cerebellum, and in most instances of tumor involving the cerebral hemispheres. It is usually normal with tumors in or near the pituitary. (2) Conditions simulating brain tumor such as subdural hematoma, brain abscess, and brain cysts. (3) Brain edema accompanying or resulting from infection, head injury, cerebral hemorrhage or thrombosis, subarachnoid hemorrhage, and many metabolic encephalopathies. (4) Interference with cerebrospinal circulation, as in internal hydrocephalus from various causes. (5) Pseudotumor cerebri, so-called benign intracranial hypertension.

Decreased pressure (below 100 mm.) is found in states of dehydration or in instances in which the spinal fluid column has been shortened as a result of block along the subarachnoid space, as in some cases of spinal cord tumor. It must be recognized that the spinal fluid pressure may also be low merely because the needle is not in free communication with the subarachnoid space.

Obstruction of normal hydrodynamics of the cerebrospinal fluid is seen in instances of blockage of the subarachnoid space due to spinal cord tumor, pachymeningitis, arachnoiditis, dislocation of a vertebra, spinal cord abscess, or any other condition that interferes with the free circulation of fluid. The technique for evaluating spinal fluid dynamics has been described above (Queckenstedt test).

APPEARANCE. The cerebrospinal fluid is normally colorless. It may be turbid because of accumulation of cells, either red or white. In cases of hemorrhage it is bloody, and the supernatant fluid is generally yellow, or xanthochromic; xanthochromia generally results from the breakdown of blood pigments but may be noted in instances of subarachnoid block and other conditions characterized by very high protein content. A so-called Froin syndrome may be evident: This consists of xanthochromia with high protein content, the spinal fluid coagulating on standing.

CELLS. The cell content of the cerebrospinal fluid is increased in so many conditions that it is impossible and pointless to enumerate them. A white cell content of more than six cells is abnormal, while red cells in any amount are of pathological significance, if they are not the result of a traumatic puncture.

Acute meningeal infections are invariably associated with cell increase, the type and number of cells depending on the cause of the meningitis. In general, acute bacterial infections result in an increase of polymorphonuclear leukocytes in the spinal fluid, whereas viral infections are associated with increase in lymphocytes (although polymorphonuclears may appear very early in the course of viral disease, as in the first few hours of infection with poliomyelitis virus). Lymphocytic pleocytosis is not restricted to viral infections of the nervous system, however, being found in chronic or granulomatous infections such as neurosyphilis or tuberculosis meningitis; in other chronic meningitides such as torula meningitis; in invasion of the meninges by neoplastic cells, as in so-called carcinomatosis and lymphomatosis of the meninges. Lymphocytes also appear in the spinal fluid during recovery from acute bacterial meningitis.

PROTEIN. An increase of protein is also found under many circumstances. It occurs in both acute and chronic meningitis, in meningeal hemorrhage, in some tumors (particularly those lying close to pial or ependymal surfaces, or in the cerebellopontine angle), in demyelinating disorders, in degenerative disease of various sorts, and in block of the spinal subarachnoid space due to cord tumor or other obstructing lesions. It may be elevated in certain diseases of spinal roots or peripheral nerves, as in the Guillain-Barré syndrome of acute "infectious" polyneuritis (albumino-cytologic dissociation), and is frequently abnormal in cases of diabetes, particularly those with neurological complications. In multiple sclerosis an increase of the gamma globulin, and particularly of the γG fraction, to above 14 per cent of the total protein is common and achieves particular diagnostic significance when the total protein content falls within the normal range. It is therefore apparent that an increase in cerebrospinal fluid protein may be found in many neurological conditions but is of specific diagnostic significance in very few. Nonetheless, an increased protein content must always be considered abnormal and when found should not be dismissed without an adequate explanation of its occurrence.

SUGAR. The sugar content of the cerebrospinal fluid may be increased or decreased and is dependent at least normally on blood sugar levels. Increase of sugar is of no diagnostic value. Decreased sugar content is found in acute bacterial meningitis, in tuberculous meningitis, and in meningeal carcinomatosis. In viral meningoencephalitis, on the other hand, the sugar is generally normal. In general, a decreased sugar content is in itself of little diagnostic significance unless accompanied by other abnormalities such as increase of cells.

CHLORIDES. Although decreased to some extent with many infections, a serious decrease in spinal fluid chloride was once thought a major if not pathognomonic feature of tuberculous meningitis. In fact, the chloride level in spinal fluid appears to follow the blood level fairly closely, and a reduction is an invariable accompaniment of the hypochloremia attendant upon recurrent vomiting and debilitation. Thus, a determination of the spinal fluid chloride is of no real diagnostic significance and has generally been discarded.

COLLOIDAL GOLD. The colloidal gold (gold-sol) curve of Lange has little diagnostic significance in most nervous diseases. It is abnormal in many, but of direct significance in few, and is commonly regarded as an indirect measurement of the level of gamma globulin. Instances of the "orthodox" patterns of the colloidal gold curve are as follows (1) first zone (paretic) curve: 5555543210; (2) second zone (tabetic) curve: 1233321000; (3) third zone (meningitic) curve: 0000012310. The greatest value of the colloidal gold curve is in neurosyphilis, particularly in general paresis, in which the paretic or first zone curve (5555543210) is found in 90 per cent of untreated cases. Such a curve, however, is not pathognomonic of paresis, being found in other forms of neurosyphilis, and at times in brain tumors and tuberculous meningitis. The colloidal gold curve is also abnormal in many cases of multiple sclerosis, and it may have diagnostic value in these circumstances. Apart from neurosyphilis and multiple sclerosis, the test has little or no specific diagnostic significance, and, as pointed out, the curve may be deranged in many other conditions. A negative colloidal gold curve (0^{10}) by no means excludes organic disease of the nervous system; a positive curve on the other hand signifies structural disease, but it gives no information in the great majority of cases as to the nature of the offending disease. Finally, it should be stressed that numerical values of up to 2 on the usual scale of 0 to 5 cannot be considered abnormal in any respect.

ELECTROENCEPHALOGRAPHY

Electroencephalography consists briefly of the amplification, recording, and analysis of the electrical potentials of the brain. The electrical activity as recorded from the usual scalp electrodes is not that of the individual neurons but represents rather a synthesis of the activity of many neurons. Neither cutaneous sensory stimulation nor the induction of motor activity alters the scalp record. The basic

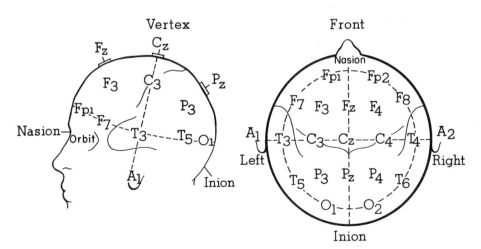

FIGURE 4-2. Standard pattern of placement of scalp electrodes for recording of routine electroencephalogram.

resting rhythm is, however, affected by opening the eyes and by alteration in attention. The electroencephalogram (EEG) must be used in conjunction with the clinical history and examination, and with other studies, for proper interpretation. There are few instances in which it has absolute value, and the diagnosis of cerebral disease by means of the EEG alone should be avoided. The EEG is a laboratory test and should be used like all other such tests. Even in epilepsy, in which it has perhaps its greatest value, it is not absolute in its diagnostic significance, and, in fact, normal or nondiagnostic EEG records occur in patients with all types of seizures. The EEG, it should be emphasized, cannot replace a careful complete clinical study.

The technique consists essentially of the application of electrodes to the scalp, with amplification and recording of the potential difference between these electrodes. In common use are solder or metal discs applied to the scalp with bentonite or

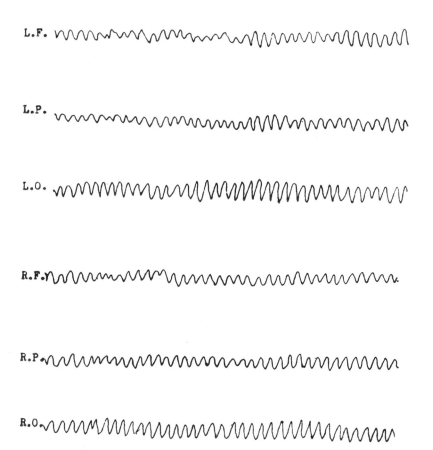

FIGURE 4-3.   Electroencephalogram, showing normal 8-10/sec. rhythm in frontal, parietal, and occipital areas of the cortex.

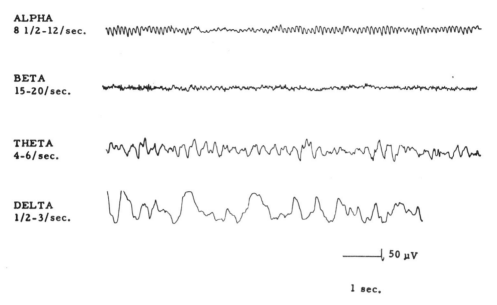

ALPHA
8 1/2-12/sec.

BETA
15-20/sec.

THETA
4-6/sec.

DELTA
1/2-3/sec.

50 μV

1 sec.

FIGURE 4-4.   Range of frequencies in the electroencephalogram.

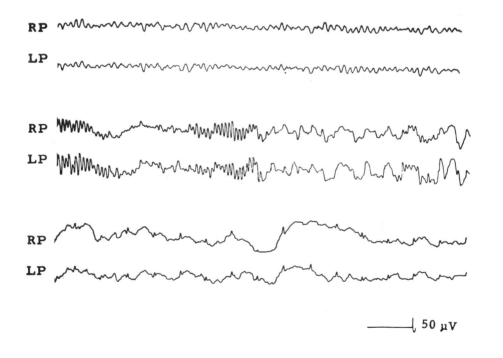

RP

LP

RP

LP

RP

LP

50 μV

1 sec.

FIGURE 4-5.   Development of sleep as seen in interrupted records from the right (RP) and left (LP) parietal leads. The irregular slight slowing and low amplitude of drowsiness giving way to 14/sec. sleep spindles, which, in turn, are followed by large slow waves.

similar paste material or fine needle electrodes inserted into the subcutaneous tissues. During the course of neurosurgical procedures, recording of direct cortical potentials (electrocorticogram, ECoG) may be used to localize abnormal discharging foci.

Electroencephalographic records are obtained over relatively long periods, thus demanding a constant, yet inexpensive, method of recording. Electromagnetic ink writers faithfully reproduce waves varying in frequency from 1 in 3 seconds to 50 a second. Amplification is necessary, since the average voltage of the cortical potentials is about 30 millionths of a volt; vacuum tubes and transistors are utilized for this purpose. While there is considerable variation from clinic to clinic in the precise location of electrodes, these are usually applied symmetrically over the frontal, parietal, occipital, and anterior and mid temporal lobes of each side, and on the ears. For special purposes, nasopharyngeal or sphenoidal electrodes are utilized. Tracings are obtained by recording the potential differences from scalp electrode to ear electrode and from scalp electrode to scalp electrode. An "indifferent" electrode may be used, especially for sleep recordings; this may be placed in the midline, usually at the base of the skull or shoulder region. The study must be carried out in a quiet room, adequately shielded against electrical artifacts. The patient must be comfortable, quiet, and relaxed, with eyes closed, but not asleep except for specific purposes as noted below.

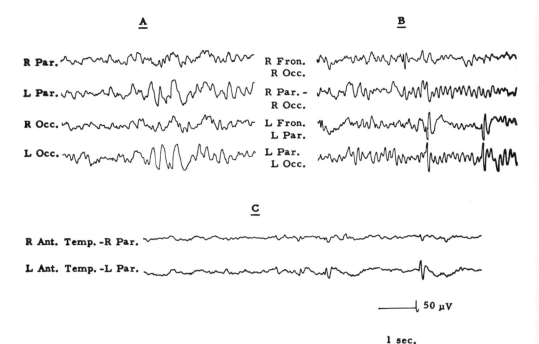

FIGURE 4-6. Focal activity in the EEG, arising spontaneously (A and B) and during sleep "activation" (C). A. High-voltage slow waves arise from the left hemisphere principally and are more pronounced in the left parietal and occipital leads. B. Sharp spike-like waves arise from the left parietal lead. During sleep (as in C) temporal lobe discharges may occur in patients with psychomotor seizures.

The most characteristic feature of normal adult records obtained under such standard resting conditions is the 8½- to 12-per-second (alpha) rhythm. This is usually seen best in occipital tracings and least in the frontal regions. At birth, frequencies of 1 to 3 per second predominate. With increasing age, the trend is toward faster frequencies, so that by 14 years of age adult-type records are obtained with some childhood features persisting. The frontal and parietal regions are not uncommonly the last to assume adult features, usually no later than 19 years of age. The electroencephalographic pattern is considered chai-acteristic for each subject, but wide variations in individual patterns are found; one such commonly encountered is of low voltage with fast frequencies in all leads. When the subject opens his eyes, a prompt decrease in amplitude of the recorded brain waves (the alerting response) ensues. The same effect is produced by mental attention, such as the computation of a difficult problem. In the early stages of sleep the 10-per-second activity becomes of lower voltage. As sleep deepens, 14-per-second to 16-per-second spindle waves appear, followed by high-voltage, slow waves with frequencies ranging from ½ to 3 per second.

Electroencephalography has been especially helpful to the clinician under two conditions: (1) in the diagnosis of epilepsy and the differential diagnosis of convulsive disorders and (2) in the localization of lesions of the cerebrum.

During epileptic seizures, certain more or less typical electroencephalographic patterns are encountered. Thus, the grand mal seizure is characterized by fast, high-voltage spikes, observed in all leads though possibly beginning with a focal or lateralizing predominance. In petit mal attacks, 3-per-second rounded waves followed or preceded by fast spikes are most frequently seen beginning and ending quite synchronously in all leads. In psychomotor seizures, spike discharges in temporal leads are usual, sometimes encountered as square-topped, 4- to 6-per-second waves. During interseizure records in epileptic patients, isolated spikes may be found; the spike discharges may occur in short groups without clinical evidence of a seizure, a "larval grand mal" attack. Short bursts of alternating waves and spikes or temporal spikes may also be encountered. In patients with petit mal epilepsy, the wave and spike may be induced by hyperventilation. In 30 to 50 per cent of epileptic patients the record between attacks is nonspecific or shows no abnormality. When the record is abnormal, the electroencephalogram may contribute to the localization of the epileptogenic site, demonstrating a focal point from which seizure activity appears to spread.

Various methods of inducing electroencephalographic abnormalities are used. Hyperventilation has already been mentioned, having long been recognized as of value in producing typical petit mal discharges. Recording during sleep may bring out abnormal discharges in all types of epilepsy, particularly in temporal lobe seizures. Carefully controlled intravenous injection of Metrazol has been found efficacious in demonstrating foci of epileptogenic activity. This may be combined with photic stimulation, or the latter may be used alone as an additional mode of activation.

Gross lesions of the cerebrum that lie within the range of the scalp electrodes may be localized by means of electroencephalography. For example, delta activity

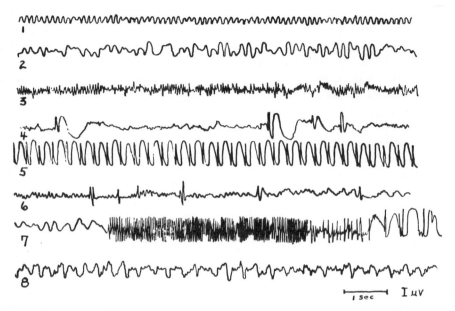

FIGURE 4-7. Normal and abnormal cerebral rhythms. 1. Normal alpha rhythm. 2. Slow irregular waves. 3. Fast waves or discharges. 4. Spike and wave, petit mal variant. 5. Spike and wave, petit mal discharge. 6. Spike discharges. 7. Grand mal discharge. 8. Psychomotor discharge at 4-6/sec. (From List, C. F., Burge, C. H., and Hodges, F. J.: Intracranial Angiography. Radiology 45:1, 1945.)

(½-per-second to 3-per-second waves of high voltage) may be found in relation to the electrode over a hemorrhage, tumor, or, most strikingly, abscess. The closer the lesion to the surface of the cerebrum, the more clear-cut and reliable is the localization; deep-seated cerebral and midline lesions are thus localized much less well than more superficial lesions. When the lesion is in the posterior fossa, little assistance is derived from the EEG in this regard.

The EEG may also be helpful in head injuries, in metabolic encephalopathies, and in assessing the depth of coma. Curiously rhythmical discharges appear in a variety of circumstances, as, for example, in so-called subacute inclusive body (sclerosing) encephalitis or in the neuronal lipidoses. At times, as with subdural hematoma, a reduction of electrical activity is of greater significance than the heightened activity to which attention is ordinarily directed. A virtually flat record is not uncommonly found in Huntington's chorea. Finally, the importance of a persistent isoelectric tracing as an indicator of brain death cannot be overestimated, particularly as regards selection of patients as donors for organ transplants.

The results of electroencephalographic study of the so-called functional psychoses—manic-depressive, schizophrenia, and involutional melancholia—are inconclusive. Thus, while there are more frequent EEG abnormalities in the total group, it is impossible to establish the presence of a psychosis, much less its type, by the record of an individual patient. Abnormalities of the electroencephalogram are more common in psychoses associated with organic brain disease. In paresis, for example, both abnormally fast and abnormally slow frequencies are found.

Attempts at correlating electroencephalographic patterns with intelligence level in feeble-minded subjects have also been unsuccessful. The greater incidence of abnormalities in those with very low intelligence is more likely correlated with the underlying cerebral disease than with the intelligence level per se.

In the field of psychiatric disorders, the greatest service has been rendered by the electroencephalogram in the study of children exhibiting behavior problems. The high incidence of abnormalities has now been well established; these are often similar to those occurring during psychomotor seizures.

MYELOGRAPHY

Pantopaque or some other hyperbaric radiopaque substance may be injected into the subarachnoid space for the purpose of creating a contrast medium against which one may visualize defects within the spinal canal. It may be introduced by the lumbar or cisternal routes, almost always the former. Injection is carried out with the patient on a fluoroscopic table in the roentgenographic room. Lumbar puncture is carried out in the usual fashion, and 10 cc. of spinal fluid is collected. Ten cubic centimeters of Pantopaque, previously warmed by immersion of the ampule in warm water, is poured into the barrel of a syringe, which is then attached to the lumbar puncture needle. The contrast material is injected slowly, from 3 to 10 cc. being utilized; for lumbar myelography, the smaller amount of dye may be adequate, but for thoracic and cervical myelography the full 10 cc. is generally required. The free flow of spinal fluid should be checked during the injection. The column of oil is observed under the fluoroscope on a tilt table, with appropriate positioning for maximal visualization of defects. Spot films are taken for a permanent record. Following full radiographic study, the Pantopaque is generally removed as completely as possible; when a complete or nearly complete block has been demonstrated, however, removal of the oil with any degree of suction may prove extremely dangerous and should be avoided.

The contrast media employed in myelography are not biologically inert, and their use is not entirely free of hazard. Meningeal irritation with frank sterile meningitis is common after use of these agents, and an increase in cellular and protein content can be documented. Local root irritation is frequent, and radicular pain may linger for some time. Rarely, adhesive arachnoiditis characterized by root pain, weakness, sensory loss, and sphincter disorder follows myelography. In an effort to avoid these side effects, *air myelography* is sometimes utilized; the technical problems associated with this variety of myelographic study are formidable, but in experienced hands it seems a very useful procedure.

In cases of complete block of the subarachnoid pathways, arrest of the contrast medium is seen. In incomplete block some of the oil escapes around the block, though its movement may be very slow. The precise configuration of the defect may be of material assistance in determining whether the offending lesion is intra-medullary or extramedullary. Errors in interpretation of apparent blockage of the oil are common, so that care must be exercised in accepting the results. False blocks are not uncommon, and tumors and other lesions blocking the subarachnoid space may not be seen in some instances. On occasion, and particularly with vascular malformations of the cord, the lesion may be missed entirely unless the patient is turned over and fluoroscopic examination made while he is lying on his back.

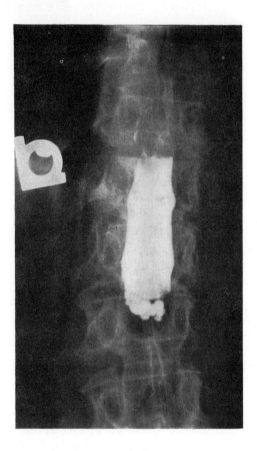

FIGURE 4-8. Pantopaque myelogram revealing complete block due to extramedullary meningioma.

In recent years myelography has found additional application in the early diagnosis of tumors of the posterior fossa, particularly acoustic neuromas, especially in cases in which other radiographic procedures have failed to document the presence of a neoplasm suspected on clinical and otologic grounds. For this purpose, Pantopaque is introduced into the lumbar sac as for ordinary myelography, but is then run up above the foramen magnum and into the cerebellopontine angles and the acoustic canals. Intracanalicular acoustic tumors less than 1 cm. in diameter can be demonstrated in this fashion.

PNEUMOENCEPHALOGRAPHY

Pneumoencephalography may be briefly defined as contrast radiography based upon the introduction of air into the subarachnoid space and ventricular system via the lumbar route. Although often a painful procedure, and one that may incapacitate a patient for several days because of severe headaches, it is quite safe in most circumstances and frequently of considerable value in the diagnosis of certain varieties of disease of the nervous system. This technique finds its widest application in atrophic and degenerative disorders and hydrocephalus, but it may also be of substantial assistance in the diagnosis of suprasellar and posterior fossa tumors (though potentially hazardous in the latter circumstance). Largely supplanted by angiography in the diagnosis of supratentorial tumors and other mass lesions, pneumoencephalography may still be of value in doubtful cases or in those with deep midline lesions. A very important contraindication to the use of pneumoencephalography is increased intracranial pressure as evidenced, for example, by papilledema. When the intracranial pressure is increased, air may be introduced directly into the ventricles from above through burr holes in the skull, a method referred to as *ventriculography*. With utilization of this form of study, visualization of the subarachnoid pathways and of the aqueduct and fourth ventricle is unfortunately much less satisfactory than with ordinary pneumoencephalography. On occasion, a radiopaque oil such as Pantopaque is introduced into the lateral ventricle through a burr hole to produce positive contrast ventriculography; this may be of great benefit when precise delineation of the aqueduct of Sylvius, fourth ventricle, and lateral recesses is required.

The pneumoencephalographic study is carried out in the roentgenographic department. The patient, previously sedated, is sitting up and straddling a chair, the arms and chin resting on a pillow thrown over the back of the chair; a specially constructed revolving chair capable of rotating in any plane is often utilized instead. Lumbar puncture is carried out in the usual fashion: Sufficient spinal fluid is ordinarily removed for routine examination (4 to 10 cc.), although on some occasions no spinal fluid at all is withdrawn. Ten cubic centimeters or less of air is then drawn through sterile gauze into a sterile syringe and injected into the subarachnoid space, after which a spot film is obtained to confirm the entrance of air into the ventricular system. An additional 10 to 30 cc. of air may then be injected in 10 cc. increments; it is not necessary to withdraw equal amounts of spinal fluid. Less air is required in infants and children than in adults. Since the normal capacity of the ventricular system is substantially less than 30 cc. in the adult, there is usually no need to employ very large quantities of air. If no air at all will enter the ventricular system despite change of position of the head, one must be very suspicious of the presence of an intracranial mass lesion and turn to other methods for diagnosis. Temperature, pulse, respiration, and blood pressure readings are obtained before the procedure is begun, and the last three are recorded every 5 or 10 minutes thereafter. If an appreciable fall in pressure ensues, caffeine sodium benzoate is given subcutaneously. Profound hypotension may necessitate cessation

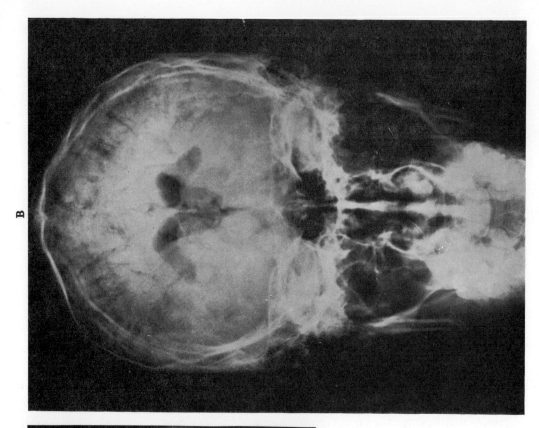

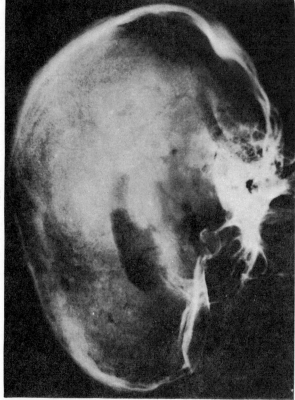

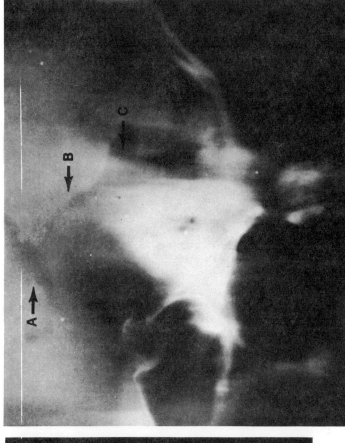

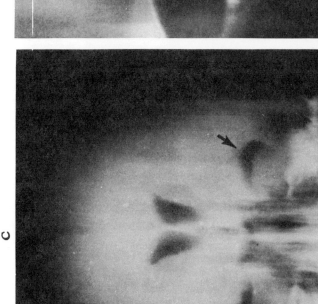

FIGURE 4-9. Normal pneumoencephalograms.

A. Lateral projection in brow-up position. The frontal horns and bodies of the lateral ventricles are well visualized; the occipital horns are not filled with air in this position. The foramen of Monro is clearly seen, and there is a small amount of air in the third ventricle. The pontine, interpeduncular, and chiasmatic cisterns are readily identified at the base.

B. Anteroposterior projection through the bodies of the lateral ventricles. The third ventricle is seen as a slit in the midline. The origin of the temporal horns is readily identified.

C. Tomogram in the anteroposterior plane, demonstrating air in the lateral and third ventricles as well as in the temporal horns (arrows).

D. Normal relationships between the posterior part of the third ventricle (A), the aqueduct of Sylvius (B), and the fourth ventricle (C) as visualized in lateral projection.

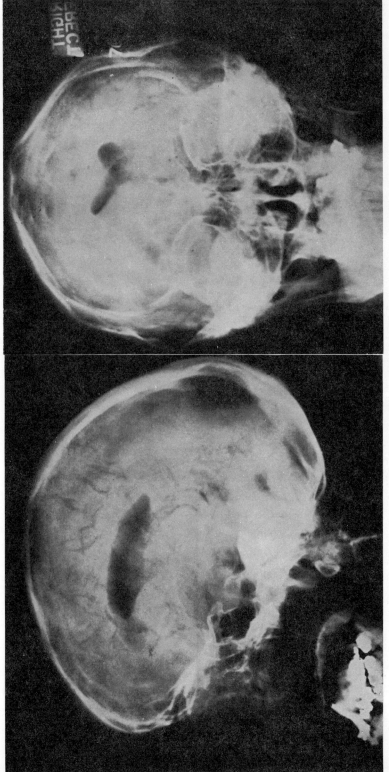

FIGURE 4-10. Pneumoencephalogram of a left frontal lobe tumor, showing encroachment on the anterior horn of the left lateral ventricle in both lateral and antero-posterior views and the shift of the midline structures to the right side.

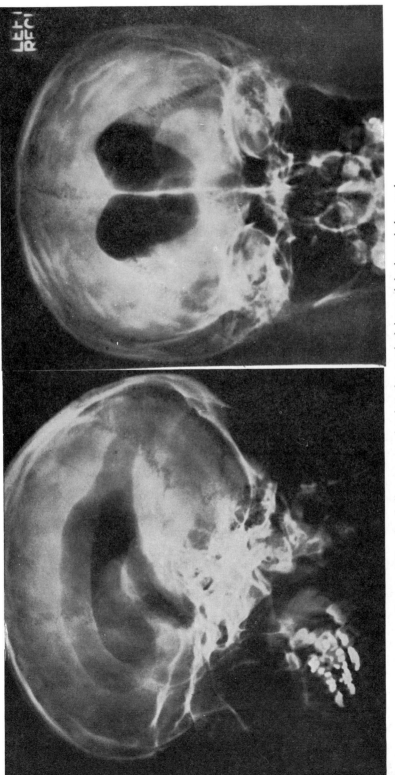

FIGURE 4-11. Cerebellar tumor, showing the marked internal hydrocephalus and the failure of filling of the fourth ventricle.

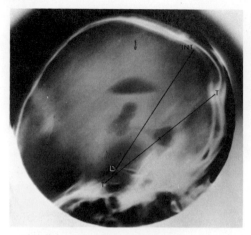

FIGURE 4-12. Methods of determining displacement of the aqueduct and fourth ventricle with pneumoencephalography. The line T-T, sometimes called Twining's line, is drawn from the tuberculum sella to the torcular Herophili; its midpoint normally falls within the fourth ventricle, usually close to the floor. The line D-INT originates on the dorsum sella and is projected through the site of junction of aqueduct and fourth ventricle to the inner table of the skull. The aqueduct ordinarily lies where the anterior and middle thirds of this line meet. Courtesy of Dr. Carlos F. Gonzalez, to whom we are also indebted for Figures 4-14, 4-15, and 4-16.

of the study. After the necessary films are taken the patient is returned to bed and placed in the Trendelenburg position for 24 hours.

In instances of tumor or other expanding lesion, distortion or obliteration of the ventricles in the vicinity of the mass is the cardinal encephalographic abnormality. The precise alteration depends of course on the specific site involved. Thus, tumors involving the cerebral hemispheres in general distort or completely obliterate the ventricle on the side of the lesion and shift the midline structures to the opposite side. The contralateral ventricle may be enlarged as a result of occlusion of the foramen of Monro. If the mass is frontal, the anterior horn of the ventricle will be encroached upon; if temporal, the temporal horn; if parietal, the body or posterior horn, etc. In third ventricle tumors the lateral ventricles are generally dilated, and changes within the third ventricle itself may be seen. Lesions in the immediate vicinity of the third ventricle, such as pinealomas, distort the air bubble in a manner in keeping with the direction of growth and compression. Tumors of the vermis of the cerebellum occlude the fourth ventricle and result in internal hydrocephalus involving the third and lateral ventricles, with distortion of the roof or complete obliteration of the fourth; the aqueduct may be displaced anteriorly as well. Cerebellopontine angle tumors may similarly demonstrate internal hydrocephalus, but much earlier encroachment upon the lateral recess of the fourth ventricle may be found. Intrinsic tumors of the brain stem may cause backward displacement of the aqueduct and fourth ventricle and obliteration of the prepontine cisterns. Incomplete filling of the chiasmatic or prechiasmatic cisterns is characteristically found with suprasellar mass lesions, and compression of the floor of the third ventricle may also be seen.

Conditions characterized by simple atrophy of brain tissue are particularly well demonstrated by pneumoencephalography. Generalized atrophy, reflected in increase in size of the entire ventricular system, may be seen in many conditions, such as Alzheimer's disease or Huntington's chorea; the ventricles are usually enlarged in a symmetrical fashion, and, as a rule, the dilatation tends to be more striking in the lateral than in the third or fourth ventricles. When ventricular enlargement develops as a result of a loss of nervous parenchyma, as in degenerative diseases of this sort, the term *hydrocephalus ex vacuo* is sometimes applied. Cerebral atrophy may also be localized, as for example with a post-traumatic meningocerebral cicatrix, and in such an instance only localized enlargement of the ventricle is found. When such focal atrophy is very marked, a frank cyst in communication with the ventricle may develop and be visualized with an air study; this is designated a *porencephalic cyst.* In the presence of a restricted atrophic process, the entire ventricular system may be distorted and shifted toward the lesion; such an *atrophic shift* is presumably a result of scarring and contraction. Atrophy of the cortical gyri themselves, either local or generalized, may also be evident with pneumoencephalography, but the significance of collections of air in the sulci may be overestimated, and the interpretation of such cortical air must be undertaken with great caution, particularly if there is no associated ventricular dilatation. Cerebellar degenerations are not uncommonly visualized by recognizable shrinkage of the folia, particularly of the superior portion of the cerebellum, along with localized enlargement of the fourth ventricle.

Arachnoiditis may also be diagnosed with an air study, particularly those instances of chiasmatic arachnoiditis characterized by failure of filling of the chiasmatic and prechiasmatic cisterns. A failure of air to enter the cortical subarachnoid spaces over the convexity of the hemispheres is sometimes taken as evidence for arachnoiditis here, but this interpretation must be accepted only with great reservation, since failure to fill the subarachnoid channels with air is often due to technical problems alone. Finally, the significance of pneumoencephalography in the diagnosis of hydrocephalus is self-evident; the importance of identifying and defining as accurately as possible the exact site of obstruction of flow of the spinal fluid cannot be overestimated.

ARTERIOGRAPHY

Cerebral angiography has largely supplanted pneumoencephalography as a prime diagnostic tool under many circumstances, particularly in the diagnosis of supratentorial mass lesions and in the evaluation of a variety of vascular diseases. It is carried out by direct injection, generally percutaneous, of a radiopaque material into the carotid or vertebral arteries, or indirectly through the aortic arch or brachial vessels. As the bolus of material is swept through the cerebral circulation a number of serial radiographs are obtained in both lateral and anteroposterior projections; depending upon equipment available, two injections of dye may be necessary for full evaluation in the two planes. Assessment of the arterial, capillary, and venous phases of the circulation is permitted, and at least a rough estimate of circulation time may be made. Although the great venous sinuses are also visualized by this technique, in some circumstances direct injection of the superior sagittal sinus itself is warranted (sinogram).

The alterations looked for with an arteriogram may be grouped into three major categories:

1. *Structural abnormalities of vessels.* Vascular malformations and aneurysms are obvious instances of this type of change. Stenotic or thrombosed vessels

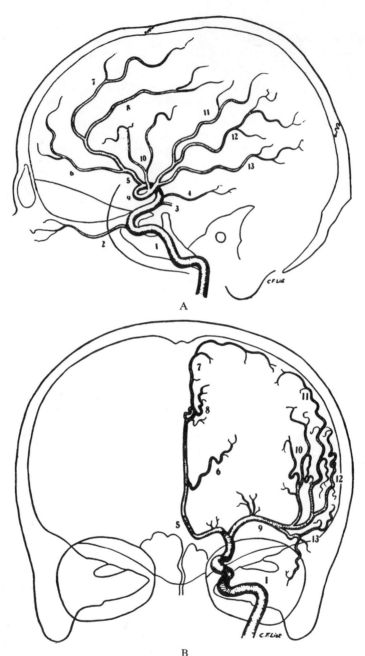

A

B

FIGURE 4-13.   Schematic drawings of normal arteriograms and venogram.
A. Carotid arteriogram, lateral projection.
B. Carotid arteriogram, anteroposterior projection.   1. Internal carotid artery.   2. Ophthalmic artery.   3. Posterior communicating artery.   4. Anterior choroidal artery.   5. Anterior cerebral artery.   6. Frontopolar artery.   7. Callosomarginal artery.   8. Pericallosal artery.   9. Middle cerebral artery.   10. Ascending frontoparietal artery.   11. Posterior parietal artery.   12. Angular artery.   13. Posterior temporal artery.

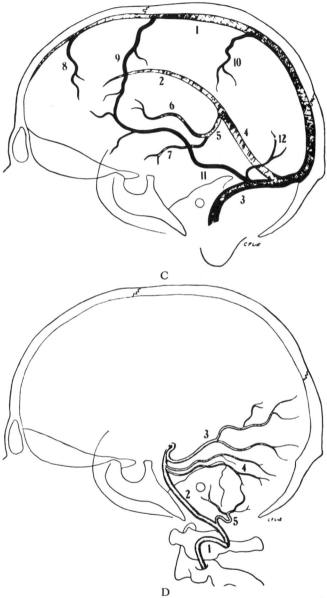

FIGURE 4-13 (continued). Schematic drawings of normal arteriograms and venogram.
C. Normal venogram, lateral projection, obtained by carotid injection. Superficial veins are shaded more darkly than sinuses and deep veins. 1. Superior sagittal sinus. 2. Inferior sagittal sinus. 3. Transverse sinus. 4. Straight sinus. 5. Great cerebral vein of Galen. 6. Internal cerebral vein. 7. Basal vein of Rosenthal. 8. Frontal ascending vein. 9. Rolandic vein of Trolard. 10. Parietal ascending vein. 11. Communicating temporal vein of Labbé. 12. Descending temporo-occipital vein.
D. Normal vertebral arteriogram, lateral projection. 1. Vertebral artery. 2. Basilar artery. 3. Posterior cerebral artery. 4. Superior cerebellar artery. 5. Posterior inferior cerebellar artery. (From List, C. F., Burge, C. H., and Hodges, F. J.: Intracranial Angiography. Radiology 45:1, 1945.)

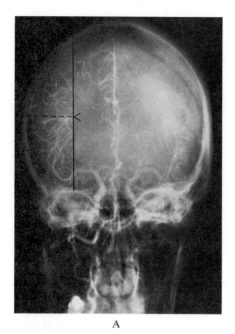

A

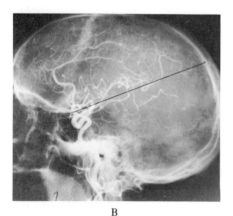

B

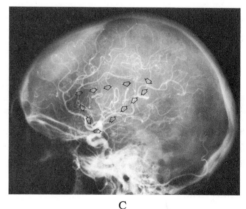

C

FIGURE 4-14. Pertinent landmarks identifiable with the carotid angiogram of use in determining the direction and degree of shift of the vascular structures as a result of intracranial disease.

A. The sylvian point (arrow), representing the mesial curving of the last major sylvian branch of the middle cerebral artery, and, thus, the posterior extent of the sylvian fissure. As found in the anteroposterior plane, it lies close to the midpoint of a line connecting the upper margin of the petrous pyramid, or of the roof of the orbit, to a horizontal line drawn tangential to the inner table of the vertex. It is usually 3.0 to 4.3 cm. from the inner table of the skull laterally.

B. The clinoparietal line. Drawn between the anterior clinoid and a point on the calvarium 9.0 cm. above the inion, this line roughly parallels the course of the middle cerebral artery; in the adult the artery falls 0.5 cm., or less, above or below.

C. The sylvian triangle. The components of this complex structure are as follows: The *top* of the triangle follows the tops of the insular loops, i.e., the loops of the insular (sylvian) branches of the middle cerebral artery; the *apex,* or posteriormost point, of the triangle is the sylvian point; the *base* comprises a line drawn from the sylvian point to the base of the first ascending insular branch of the middle cerebral artery; the remaining *side* is equivalent to the anterior insular line, running from the origin of the first ascending insular branch to the most anterosuperior insular loop.

may be identified, and under special circumstances, such as subarachnoid hemorrhage due to rupture of an aneurysm, spasm of vessels may be encountered. Collections of abnormal vessels may be demonstrated within certain neoplasms, in particular gliomas, meningiomas, and metastatic carcinomas, and may be responsible for a so-called tumor *blush* or *stain*.

2. *Alterations in position of vessels.* Mass lesions commonly produce displacement of vessels. Such displacement may be local, and result in more or less complete and direct delineation of the mass, or distant and indirect; examples of the latter include shift of the anterior cerebral artery with anteriorly placed lesions or of the internal cerebral vein with more posteriorly placed lesions. At times such a shift or displacement of vessels is associated with a stain or blush (see above); in other instances, as with subdural hematoma, only the shift is recognized, the lesion itself being represented by an avascular area. In cases of increased intracranial pressure, as with internal hydrocephalus, the vessels may be observed to be stretched out over the dilated ventricular system.

3. *Alterations in flow patterns.* Changes in the circulatory pattern may be evident as an expression of abnormal vascular shunts, as with arteriovenous malformations or in some tumors. Collateral flow patterns may be identified in instances of thrombosis of major arteries as, for example, through the ophthalmic artery in instances of carotid artery occlusion; diminution or absence of flow is of course found distal to the site of vascular occlusion itself. A general slowing of the circulation may be noted when the intracranial pressure is elevated, for whatever reason.

Much confusion prevails concerning the specific indications for selecting either angiography or pneumoencephalography in a given patient. Briefly, it may be stated that angiography is the procedure of choice if one is concerned with the possibility of neoplasm, particularly supratentorial in location; subdural hematoma or other expanding lesions such as abscess or intracranial hematoma, particularly if associated with increasing intracranial pressure; vascular malformation or aneurysm; and stenosis, thrombosis, or other lesions of vessel wall or lumen. Despite a definite, though low, morbidity rate, angiography possesses the virtue of leaving unchanged cerebral hydrodynamic mechanisms, and is thus of relative safety when the intracranial pressure is elevated. Pneumoencephalography, on the other hand, is the procedure of choice in the delineation of degenerative and atrophic processes and in the evaluation of hydrocephalus. The application of this procedure to neoplasms, particularly those in the posterior fossa, is potentially hazardous but in skilled hands is often of paramount importance. Deep midline tumors, particularly those in the vicinity of the pituitary fossa, may also require pneumoencephalography for accurate diagnosis, as do intraventricular neoplasms and cysts. Further, in the evaluation of a neurological problem such as a seizure disorder without clear-cut focal or lateralizing signs, pneumoencephalography is the contrast study of choice initially. Finally, it should be emphasized that angiography and pneumoencephalography are not mutually exclusive procedures. Both may be, and often are, utilized in the same patient for purposes of accurate diagnosis of neurological illness.

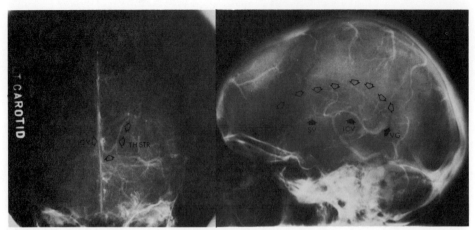

FIGURE 4-15. Useful landmarks apparent during the venous phase of the carotid angiogram.
A. The internal cerebral vein (ICV), as demonstrated in the anteroposterior plane, an important deep midline landmark. The course of the thalamostriate vein (THSTR) is also indicated (arrows); conclusions as to the presence of significant ventricular enlargement or distortion may be drawn from identification of deviations in this vessel's course.
B. The outline of the lateral ventricles. The floor of the ventricle is delineated by the septal (SV) and internal cerebral (ICV) veins and the vein of Galen (VG); the ventricular roof is marked by the terminal portions of the periependymal, e.g., anterior and posterior caudate, veins (arrows). Enlargement of the ventricles can be readily identified with angiography if this outline is recognized.

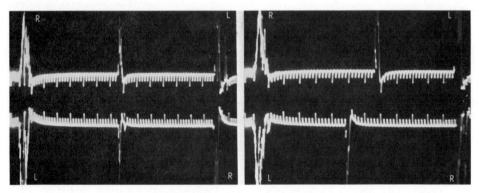

FIGURE 4-16.   Echoencephalogram. Left: Normal tracing. Right: Deviation
of midline (falx) from right to left.

BRAIN SCANNING

Radioisotope (scintillation) scanning provides a safe screening procedure in the diagnosis of intracranial lesions, and one which is generally utilized before resorting to contrast studies. A variety of isotopes has been employed for this type of study, originally I^{131}-labeled diiodofluorescein and I^{131}-labeled serum albumin, and more recently Hg^{203}-labeled chlormerodrin and technetium^{99m}. Offering safety and relative ease of performance, scanning techniques designed to delineate abnormal areas of isotope concentration find their greatest application in the recognition of supratentorial lesions, particularly neoplasms. Because of overlying extracranial muscle masses, which may mask subjacent concentrations of the isotope, scans are much less informative with lesions at the base of the skull, as in the vicinity of the sella, and in the posterior fossa. It must be emphasized that not all areas of increased concentration necessarily represent neoplasm. Uptake of isotope may also be noted in the course of a softening, and comparative follow-up studies may be necessary if clinical suspicion of tumor remains high. Intracranial hematomas are frequently demonstrated with this technique as well, and vascular malformations may be dramatically manifested. Lacerations and hematomas of the scalp may also concentrate the isotope, leading to occasional errors in diagnosis.

So-called RISA (radioiodinated serum albumin) cisternography comprises another isotope scanning procedure of value, particularly in instances of occult (normotensive) hydrocephalus and in other conditions in which a dynamic presentation of the flow of cerebrospinal fluid may be informative. The isotope is injected into the lumbar subarachnoid space, then followed by serial scanning as it enters the subarachnoid cisterns at the base of the brain, migrates over the convexities of the cerebral hemispheres, and finally enters the superior sagittal sinus. In cases of obstruction of flow over the convexities, as due for example to an incisural block, the isotope lingers for protracted periods within the cisterns, not uncommonly concentrates in large quantities within the ventricles themselves, and traverses the cerebral subarachnoid pathways only with considerable delay.

ECHOENCEPHALOGRAPHY

Like brain scanning, echoencephalography comprises a safe diagnostic procedure commonly utilized as part of a preliminary screening in the search for intracranial disease. Utilizing ultrasonic techniques and the recording of echoes derived from deep structures within the skull, this procedure is most valuable in identifying the midline and, thus, in documenting a shift of the cranial contents from one side to the other in expanding lesions such as subdural hematoma. Experienced investigators may also satisfactorily demonstrate the contour of the ventricular system and even the thickness of intracranial hematomas under certain circumstances with this technique.

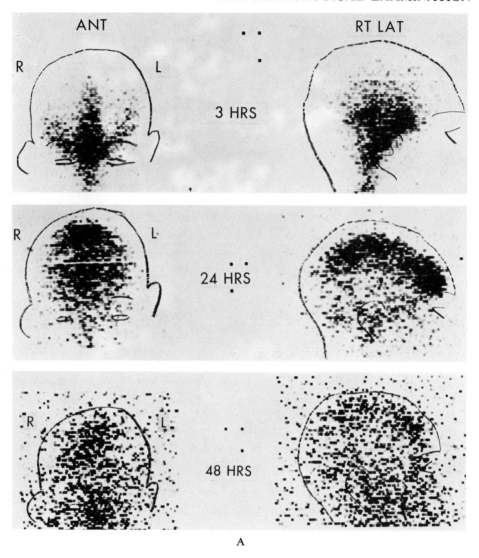

FIGURE 4-17. RISA cisternography. A. Normal series at 3, 24, and 48 hours after introduction of the isotope into the lumbar subarachnoid space. RISA is present in the basal cisterns and to some extent the ventricles at 3 hours but has largely migrated to the convexity of the hemispheres by 24 hours. Only a small amount of isotope is present at 48 hours.

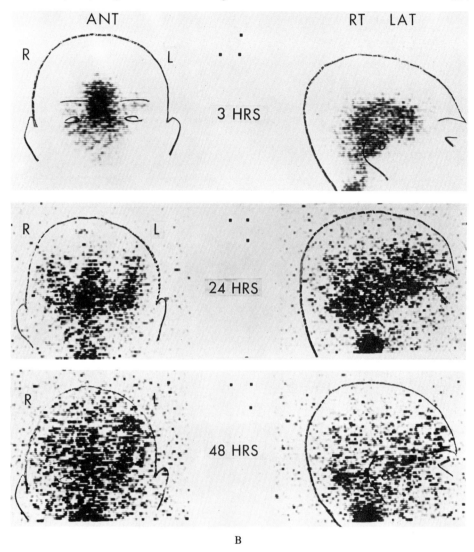

B

B. Occult (normotensive) hydrocephalus. Marked delay in migration of the isotope is observed. A strong concentration is still evident within the basal cisterns and ventricles at 24 hours, with virtually none over the convexities. Even at 48 hours a substantial amount of isotope remains concentrated within the ventricles. (Courtesy of Dr. Millard Croll.)

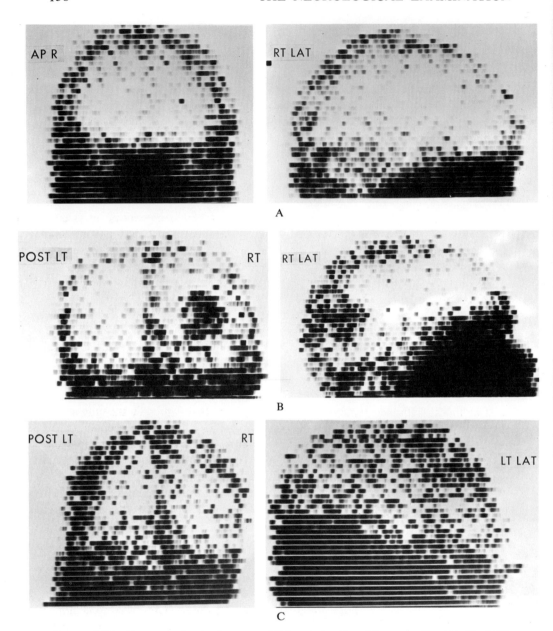

FIGURE 4-18.   Representative brain scans utilizing technetium 90 m. A. Normal. B. Astro-cytoma, evidencing dense uptake of isotope in right cerebral hemisphere posteriorly. C. Sub-dural hematoma, with prominent peripheral concentration of isotope overlying the left hemisphere. (Courtesy of Dr. Millard Croll.)

ELECTROMYOGRAPHY

Electromyography consists essentially of the observation and recording of electrical potentials derived from or arising within individual muscle fibers, such potentials being initially detected by needle electrodes, amplified electronically, and ultimately displayed on an oscilloscope or at times through a loudspeaker. Various photographic and electronic techniques permit storage of permanent records. In the normal, and in a number of disease states, a variety of individually identifiable potentials can be recognized, whose principal characteristics may be summarized as follows:

When the needle electrode is originally placed within the muscle, *insertion activity* appears, comprising potentials evoked by injury to the muscle fiber; at times nerve potentials and miniature end-plate potentials (sometimes referred to as end-plate noise) appear at this time as well. When insertional activity has subsided and the needle movement ceased, and the muscle remains at repose, spontaneously arising potentials may appear in certain pathological states. These include: (1) *Positive sharp waves,* nonpropagated potentials that vary in amplitude from 50 to 4000 microvolts with a duration of 10 milliseconds or more. Needle movement may stimulate the appearance of these potentials. Positive sharp waves are not ordinarily found in the normal; their appearance is most suggestive of denervation. (2) *Fibrillation potentials,* consisting of short duration diphasic or triphasic waves occurring at rates of 2 to 20 per second and varying in amplitude from 20 to 300 microvolts. These are commonly, although not invariably, associated with denervation or with inflammatory muscle diseases. (3) *Fasciculation potentials,* large and at times rhythmical potentials of varying form that represent the summation of a number of individual motor unit potentials. Characteristically encountered in motor system disease, fasciculation potentials may also be seen in hyperthyroidism, in uremia, in the syndrome of benign myokymia, and, on occasion, in normal individuals. (4) *Myotonic discharges,* high-frequency discharges occurring in trains of potentials and appearing particularly with electrode movement. Rates of up to 150 per second may be found; typically there is a rapid rise and a nearly as rapid fall in frequency; over the loudspeaker, these potential sequences cause a rising and falling sound reminiscent of that of a dive bomber.

After a careful search has been made for such spontaneous electrical activity, volitional movements are undertaken to elicit true action potentials. Isolated action potentials are best studied with minimal voluntary contractions; they appear as diphasic or triphasic waves of 4- to 10-millisecond duration and varying in amplitude from 300 microvolts to 2 millivolts. With increasing voluntary activity, individual action potentials build up, ultimately with maximal effort fusing in a so-called *interference pattern.* Response of the pattern of action potentials to repetitive stimulation of the muscle is also investigated, deviations from normal being encountered, for example, in myasthenia gravis, in which decay in amplitude of successive potentials is seen, and in the Lambert-Eaton syndrome, the "myasthenic" syndrome of carcinoma of the lung, in which the opposite pertains, at least with rapid stimulation.

It must be emphasized that no pattern of muscle action potential is necessarily specific for, or pathognomonic of, any particular disease. *Myopathic* illnesses generally do, however, tend to share certain electromyographic features, although some variability may be found. Insertion activity is commonly normal or nearly so; in rapidly evolving disorders such as polymyositis there may be considerable increase in insertion activity, whereas when there has been extensive replacement of muscle by fat or connective tissue, as in the late stages of dystrophy, insertional activity may be severely reduced or absent. During complete relaxation no electrical activity can be recorded in the majority of myopathies. In myotonic dystrophy, however, and in the other myotonias, post-contraction fibrillation activity is found, consisting of brief showers of small-amplitude very rapid diphasic or triphasic spike potentials presumably representing abnormally persistent activity of individual muscle fibers. In addition, as noted above, myotonic states are characterized by the presence of high-frequency discharges elicited by movement of the electrode, the so-called myotonic discharges. (These features, it should be added, permit identification of myopathies exhibiting myotonia as distinct from other disorders of muscle.) With voluntary contraction the expected build-up of action potentials with development of an interference pattern resulting from the fusion of individual potentials appears and is normal in most myopathies. Characteristically, however, one encounters rapid and low-amplitude potentials. Polyphasic potentials (so-called disintegrated or *myopathic potentials*), absent in the normal, are common with myopathy and are of major diagnostic importance.

In *denervated* muscle, electrical changes are observed that differ markedly from those of myopathy. At rest, spontaneous fibrillation potentials are common, and these small rapid potentials may be so prominent as to replace normal insertional activity. Fasciculation potentials may appear; as noted, these are most striking with disease of the anterior horn cells. The large-amplitude slow positive potentials called positive sharp waves are also characteristically found with denervation. With voluntary contraction, faulty formation of an interference pattern is seen in denervated muscle, reflecting reduction in the number of available motor units. Polyphasic potentials may also be seen but tend to be only a minor part of the electromyographic constellation of denervation. Electromyographic studies in denervation thus yield substantially different results from those in myopathy, and it is in distinguishing the two that such electrophysiological techniques achieve their most widespread application.

Among other available electrodiagnostic studies, determination of nerve conduction velocity is perhaps the most valuable. Techniques are available to assess conduction in both motor and sensory nerves. Although there is considerable variation in published conduction rates, it is apparent that with the exception of the very young, in whom conduction of the nerve impulse proceeds much more slowly than in the adult, a figure of 40 meters per second may be taken as the minimal acceptable figure for rate of conduction in a normal peripheral nerve. Nerve conduction studies find widest application in the evaluation of disorders of the peripheral nervous system but may prove of some limited value in diseases of the spinal roots and of the spinal cord itself. In instances of peripheral neuropathy, a very marked

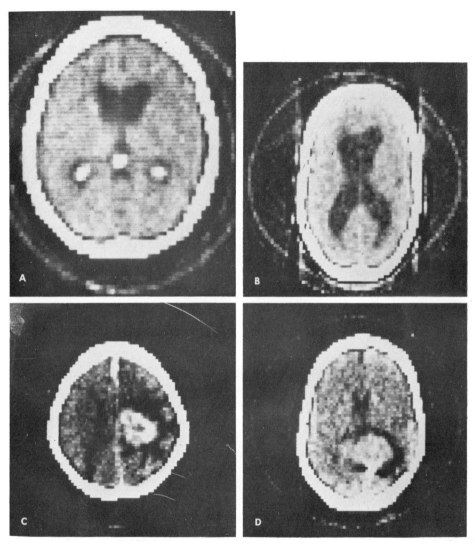

FIGURE 4-19. Representative examples of computerized transaxial tomography (EMI-scan). A, Normal scan. The principle components of the ventricular system are readily identified. The calcified pineal, with a density approximating that of the skull, is found in the midline; calcification in the choroid plexus is present bilaterally more laterally placed in the trigone. B, Hydrocephalus. There is striking symmetric enlargement of the entire ventricular system. C, Metastatic carcinoma involving the thalamus on the right. Reduced tissue density through much of the right hemisphere indicates massive edema. The center of the tumor is necrotic. D. Meningioma arising posteriorly at the junction of falx and tentorium. Radiolucent low density area surrounding the mass marks a zone of edema.

slowing in conduction velocity, in the range of 12 to 18 meters per second, suggests a demyelinating (segmental, Gombault) type of neuropathy, whereas a minimal reduction, i.e., to 30 to 40 meters per second, is more in keeping with an axonal (wallerian) type of neuropathy.

COMPUTERIZED TRANSAXIAL TOMOGRAPHY

Recently an additional radiographic tool, computerized transaxial tomography, has become available. Generally utilizing the so-called EMI scanner, this technique has in a very short time become a major and at times remarkably dramatic addition to the neurodiagnostic armamentarium. Based on computer processing of data derived from tomographic "slices" of the cranium, it permits identification of a wide range of both normal and pathological structures (Fig. 4-19) by virtue of differences in tissue density, without recourse to contrast studies (although under some circumstances the intravenous use of contrast media affords image enhancement). With this procedure, there is no appreciable hazard to the patient, and it may be used as a relatively safe screening method suitable for out-patient application. A variety of lesions may be demonstrated with clarity, for example, intra-axial and extra-axial tumors, infarcts, cysts, intracerebral and extracerebral hematomas, and inflammatory lesions. Edematous areas may be rendered in striking fashion. The size of the cortical mantle and, even more importantly, the size, shape and position of the ventricles can be assessed directly. As a result, this technique has become especially useful in the evaluation of hydrocephalus. Finally, modification and extension of this basic technique to soft tissues elsewhere in the body has been proposed.

BIBLIOGRAPHY

A Definition of Irreversible Coma. Report of the Ad Hoc Committee of the Harvard Medical School to Examine the Definition of Brain Death. JAMA 205:337, 1968.

Bender, M. B. (ed.): The Approach to Diagnosis in Modern Neurology. Grune & Stratton, New York, 1967.

Croll, M. N., Brady, L. W., Faust, D. S., Kazem, I., Antoniades, J., and Tatem, H. R., III: Comparison Brain Scanning with Mercury 203 and Technetium[99]m. Radiology 90:747, 1968.

Davidoff, L. M., and Dyke, C. G.: The Normal Encephalogram. Lea & Febiger, Philadelphia, 1951.

Davidoff, L. M., and Epstein, B. S.: The Abnormal Pneumoencephalogram. Lea & Febiger, Philadelphia, 1955.

Di Chiro, G.: An Atlas of Detailed Normal Pneumoencephalographic Anatomy. Charles C Thomas, Springfield, Ill., 1961.

Downie, A. W.: Studies in Nerve Conduction, Chapter 26 in Walton, J. N. (ed.): Disorders of Voluntary Muscle, ed. 2. Little, Brown and Co., Boston, 1969.

Gibbs, F. A., and Gibbs, E. L.: Atlas of Electroencephalography. Addison-Wesley Publishing Company, Reading, Mass., 1950-1964, vol. 1-3.

Gonzalez, C., Kricheff, I. I., Lin, J. P., and Lorber, S.: Evaluation of the Vlahovitch System for the Measurement of the Sylvian Triangle with Computer Analysis of the Results. Radiology 94:535, 1970.

Gutterman, P., and Shenkin, H. A.: Cerebral Scans in Completed Strokes: Value in Prognosis of Clinical Course. JAMA 207:145, 1969.

Hill, D., and Parr, G.: Electroencephalography: A Symposium on Its Various Aspects. Macmillan Co., New York, 1963.

Kiloh, L. G., and Osselton, J. W.: Clinical Electroencephalography, ed 2. Butterworth & Co., London, 1966.

Lenman, J. A. R., and Ritchie, A. E.: Clinical Electromyography. Pitman Medical and Scientific Publishing Co., London, 1970.

Lennox, W. G.: Epilepsy and Related Disorders. Little, Brown and Co., Boston, 1960, 2 vol.

Richardson, A. T., and Barwick, D. D.: Clinical Electromyography, Chapter 27 in Walton, J. N. (ed.): Disorders of Voluntary Muscle, ed. 2. Little, Brown and Co., Boston, 1969.

Robertson, E. G.: Pneumoencephalography. Charles C Thomas, Springfield, Ill., 1967.

Scanlan, R. L.: Positive Contrast Medium (Iophendylate) in Diagnosis of Acoustic Neuroma. Arch. Otolaryng. 80:698, 1964.

Schneck, S. A., and Claman, H. N.: CSF Immunoglobulins in Multiple Sclerosis and Other Neurological Diseases. Arch. Neurol. 20:132, 1969.

Silverman, D., Saunders, M. G., Schwab, R. S., and Masland, R. L.: Cerebral Death and the Electroencephalogram. JAMA 209:1505, 1969.

Taveras, J. M., and Wood, E. H.: Diagnostic Neuroradiology. Williams & Wilkins Co., Baltimore, 1964.

Toole, J. F. (ed.): Special Techniques for Neurologic Diagnosis. F. A. Davis Co., Philadelphia, 1969.

Tow, D. E., Wagner, H. N., DeLand, F. H., and North, W. A.: Brain Scanning in Cerebral Vascular Disease. JAMA 207:105, 1969.

Wickbom, I.: Angiography of the Carotid Artery, Parts 1 and 2. Acta Radiol. Suppl. 72. Stockholm, 1948.

Davis, D. O., and Pressman, B. D.: Computerized Tomography of the Brain. Radiol. Clin. North Am. 12:297, 1974.

Ledley, R. S., DiChiro, G., Luessenhop, A. J., and Twigg, H. L.: Computerized Transaxial X-ray Tomography of the Human Body. Science 186:207, 1974.

New, P. F. J., Scott, W. R., Schnur, J. A., Davis, K. R., and Taveras, J. M.: Computerized Axial Tomography with the EMI Scanner. Radiology 110:109, 1974.

Index

165